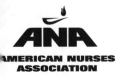

AMERICAN NURSES ASSOCIATION

D1597519

Scope AND **Standards** OF PRACTICE

Intellectual and Developmental Disabilities Nursing

SECOND EDITION

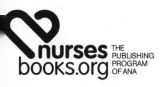

nurses books.org THE PUBLISHING PROGRAM OF ANA

American Nurses Association
Silver Spring, MD
2013

Library of Congress Cataloging-in-Publication data

Intellectual and developmental disabilities nursing : scope and standards of practice. -- 2nd ed.

p. ; cm.

Authors include Wendy M. Nehring, et al.

Rev. ed. of: Intellectual and developmental disabilities nursing / Nursing Division of the American Association on Mental Retardation. 2004.

Includes bibliographical references and index.

ISBN 978-1-55810-466-2 (soft cover)—ISBN 978-1-55810-467-9 (ebook, PDF format)—ISBN 978-1-55810-468-6 (ebook, EPUB format)—ISBN 978-1-55810-469-3 (ebook, Mobipocket format)

    I. Nehring, Wendy M., 1957- II. American Nurses Association. III. American Association on Mental Retardation. Nursing Division. Intellectual and developmental disabilities nursing.
[DNLM: 1. Developmental Disabilities—nursing. 2. Intellectual Disability—nursing. 3. Clinical Competence—standards. 4. Psychiatric Nursing—methods. 5. Psychiatric Nursing—standards. WY 160]

616.85'880231--dc23

2012038859

The American Nurses Association (ANA) is a national professional association. This joint ANA publication (*Intellectual and Developmental Disabilities Nursing: Scope and Standards of Practice, 2nd Edition*) reflects the thinking of the practice specialty of intellectual and developmental disabilities nursing on various issues and should be reviewed in conjunction with state board of nursing policies and practices. State law, rules, and regulations govern the practice of nursing, while *Intellectual and Developmental Disabilities Nursing: Scope and Standards of Practice, 2nd Edition* guides nurses in the application of their professional skills and responsibilities.

American Nurses Association
8515 Georgia Avenue, Suite 400
Silver Spring, MD 20910-3492
1-800-274-4ANA
http://www.NursingWorld.org

Published by Nursesbooks.org
The Publishing Program of ANA
http://www.Nursesbooks.org/

ISBN-13: 978-1-55810-466-2   SAN: 851-3481   03/2013

First printing: March 2013

Contents

Contributors

The nursing members of the Health and Wellness Action Group of the American Association on Intellectual and Developmental Disabilities (AAIDD) and the American Nurses Association (ANA) would like to personally thank those who contributed their valuable time and talents to *Intellectual and Developmental Disabilities Nursing: Scope and Standards of Practice, Second Edition*. The previous editions were entitled *Intellectual and Developmental Disabilities Nursing: Scope and Standards of Practice* and *Statement on the Scope and Standards for the Nurse Who Specializes in Developmental Disabilities and/or Mental Retardation* in the original edition. The terminology has changed over the years and is reflected in each edition of the scope statement and standards of practice.

The authors of *Intellectual and Developmental Disabilities Nursing: Scope and Standards of Practice, Second Edition*, include:

Wendy M. Nehring, RN, PhD, FAAN, FAAIDD

Deborah Natvig, RN, PhD

Cecily L. Betz, RN, PhD, FAAN

Teresa Savage, RN, PhD

Marilyn Krajicek, RN, EdD, FAAN

Carolyn Graff, RN, PhD, FAAIDD

Dalice Hertzberg, RN, MSN, FNP-C

Dedication of This Edition

This edition is dedicated to the memory of author Dalice Hertzberg, MSN, RN, FNP-C.

ANA Staff

Carol Bickford, PhD, RN-BC, CPHIMS—Content editor

Maureen E. Cones, Esq.—Legal counsel

Yvonne Daley Humes, MSA—Project coordinator

Eric Wurzbacher, BA—Project editor

Endorsing Organizations

The American Nurses Association has approved and acknowledges *Intellectual and Developmental Disabilities Nursing: Scope and Standards of Practice, Second Edition,* as defined herein. Approval is valid for five (5) years from the first date of publication of this document or until a new scope of practice has been approved, whichever occurs first.

About the American Nurses Association

The American Nurses Association (ANA) is the only full-service professional organization representing the interests of the nation's 3.1 million registered nurses through its constituent/state nurses associations and its organizational affiliates. The ANA advances the nursing profession by fostering high standards of nursing practice, promoting the rights of nurses in the workplace, projecting a positive and realistic view of nursing, and by lobbying the Congress and regulatory agencies on health care issues affecting nurses and the public.

About Nursesbooks.org, the Publishing Program of ANA

Nursesbooks.org publishes books on ANA core issues and programs, including ethics, leadership, quality, specialty practice, advanced practice, and the profession's enduring legacy. Best known for the foundational documents of the profession on nursing ethics, scope and standards of practice, and social policy, Nursesbooks.org is the publisher for the professional, career-oriented nurse, reaching and serving nurse educators, administrators, managers, and researchers as well as staff nurses in the course of their professional development.

Overview of the Content

Foundational Documents of Professional Nursing and Intellectual and Developmental Disabilities Nursing

The American Nurses Association (ANA) has been the vanguard for nursing practice for more than a century. *Code of Ethics for Nurses with Interpretive Statements* (ANA, 2001), *Nursing: Scope and Standards of Practice* (2nd ed., ANA, 2010a), and *Nursing's Social Policy Statement: The Essence of the Profession* (3rd ed., ANA, 2010b) are all documents produced by the ANA to inform the thinking and decision-making of registered nurses practicing in the United States and guide their practice. First, *Code of Ethics for Nurses with Interpretive Statements* (ANA, 2001) lists the nine succinct provisions that establish the ethical framework for registered nurses across all roles, levels, and settings. Second, *Nursing's Social Policy Statement: The Essence of the Profession* (ANA, 2010b) conceptualizes nursing practice, describes the social context of nursing, and provides the definition of nursing. *Nursing: Scope and Standards of Practice* (2nd ed., ANA, 2010a) outlines the expectations of the professional role of the registered nurse. It states the Scope of Nursing Practice and presents the Standards of Professional Nursing Practice and their accompanying competencies. These documents are intended to provide the public with assurances of safe and competent nursing care.

Along with these documents, specialty nursing organizations have worked with the ANA to publish specific standards of care and professional practice in their specialty. This document, concerning the care of individuals with intellectual and developmental disabilities (hereafter referred to as IDD), is a revision of *Intellectual and Developmental Disabilities Nursing: Scope and Standards of Practice* (ANA & Nursing Division of the American Association on Mental Retardation, 2004). This document has been revised to: (a) capture the changing practice of nursing in this specialty (i.e., encompassing all levels of education and all system levels of care from the individual to the system itself), (b) emphasize the unique health care needs and characteristics of individuals of all ages with IDD, and (c) incorporate the ANA standards mentioned earlier (ANA, 2010a). The last edition of these specialty standards and scope of practice is found in Appendix A. Prior to this document, the initial standards document for this specialty was entitled *Statement on the Scope and Standards for the Nurse Who Specializes in Developmental Disabilities and/or Mental Retardation* (Nursing Division of the American Association on Mental Retardation and American Nurses Association, 1998). The titles changed for each edition due to the changing acceptable terminology for the population served.

In addition, adolescents and adults with IDD and their families/legal guardians collaborate with health care professionals in making person-centered decisions about their health care. This self-advocacy has arisen in tandem with an evolving healthcare system that may or may not optimize healthcare options for all people. Therefore, in response to these changes, individuals of all ages with IDD and their families/legal guardians should be assured of safe and effective nursing care. This document addresses this care.

Additional Content

This document should also be used in conjunction with other standards of care and professional performance developed by other specialty nursing groups [e.g., *Pediatric Nursing: Scope and Standards of Practice* (Society of Pediatric Nurses, National Association of Pediatric Nurse Practitioners, & ANA, 2008); *Genetics-Genomics Nursing: Scope and Standards of Practice* (International Society of Nurses in Genetics, Inc. & ANA, 2006); *Public Health Nursing: Scope and Standards of Practice* (ANA, 2007b); *Psychiatric-Mental Health Nursing: Scope and Standards of Practice* (American Psychiatric Nurses Association, International Society of Psychiatric-Mental Health Nurses, & ANA, 2007); and *School Nursing: Scope and Standards of Practice* (2nd ed., National Association of School Nurses & ANA, 2011)]. Additional important nursing documents that address the history and context of nursing standards include *Nursing: Scope and Standards of Practice* (2nd ed., ANA, 2010a), ANA's *Principles of*

Environmental Health for Nursing Practice (ANA, 2007a), *Professional Role Competence: ANA Position Statement* (ANA, 2008), and "The Development of Foundational Nursing Documentation and Professional Nursing" (Appendix C) in *Nursing: Scope and Standards of Practice* (ANA, 2010a).

Audience for This Publication

Nurses, of any educational level and employed in any setting that serves individuals of any age with IDD, make up the primary audience for this book. Legislators, regulators, legal counsel, and the judiciary system will also want to reference it. Agencies, organizations, nurse administrators, other nurses not working in this specialty, and other interprofessional colleagues will find this an invaluable reference. In addition, healthcare consumers with IDD, their family/legal guardians, communities, and populations using healthcare and nursing services that cover the care of persons with IDD can use this document to better understand the role and responsibilities of registered nurses and advanced practice nurses who specialize in intellectual and developmental disabilities.

Scope of Intellectual and Developmental Disabilities (IDD) Nursing Practice

Nurses who specialize in intellectual and developmental disabilities (IDD) are unique in the population that they serve. Because the history of this nursing specialty was primarily institutional until the late 1950s, and because of the stigma attached to this population, many nurses have not become familiar with this area. In fact, this nursing specialty was only recognized as such by the American Nurses Association in 1997 (Nehring, 1999). Unlike many nursing specialties, the scope of practice for nurses who specialize in IDD extends across all levels of care and all health care and many educational settings. Even though healthcare consumers with IDD are present today in all communities and health care settings, they remain a vulnerable population. This is because they often require assistance to advocate for their needs and many health care professionals are not educated and skilled to care for their specific condition and developmental needs. Such health disparities were highlighted in the Surgeon General's report, *Closing the Gap: A National Blueprint for Improving the Health of Persons with Mental Retardation* (U.S. Public Health Service, 2002). Working in an interdisciplinary context, nurses continue to strive to promote the importance of the discipline of nursing in this specialty field and to provide specific health care at both the generalist and advanced practice level.

Definition of Nursing

Nursing's Social Policy Statement: The Essence of the Profession (ANA, 2010b, p. 3) builds on previous work and provides the following contemporary definition of nursing:

> *Nursing is the protection, promotion, and optimization of health and abilities, prevention of illness and injury, alleviation of suffering through the diagnosis and treatment of human response, and advocacy in the care of individuals, families/legal guardians, communities, and populations.*

This definition serves as the foundation for the following expanded description of the Scope of Nursing Practice and the Standards of Professional Nursing Practice for nurses who specialize in intellectual and developmental disabilities.

Definition of Intellectual and Developmental Disability (IDD)

Intellectual and developmental disability is a broad term that refers to a wide variety of mental and/or physical conditions that interfere with an individual's ability to function effectively at an expected developmental level. These conditions have been referred to as *developmental disabilities* or *mental retardation* in the past. Today, *intellectual and developmental disability* is the term used to describe these conditions. An intellectual and developmental disability is:

> *A disability characterized by significant limitations both in intellectual functioning and in adaptive behavior, which covers many everyday social and practical skills. This disability originates before the age of 18* (Schalock, Borthwick-Duffy, Bradley, Buntinx, Coulter, Craig, et al., 2010).

Nurses who specialize in the care of persons of all ages with IDD care for persons with these conditions. These conditions may be organic and nonorganic or social in nature.

It is important to clarify that IDD is different from chronic conditions or illness and disabilities in general. *Chronic* can simply mean any condition that exists over a period of time. Although IDD exists across time, the definition is more specific. This is also true for *disabilities*, a general term that refers to any condition that limits activities of daily living. Again, IDD may limit activities of daily living, but the conditions require understanding of more specific information regarding physiology, epidemiology, etiology, pathophysiology, genetics, diagnosis, treatment and management, follow-up, and nursing implications. The care of healthcare consumers with IDD most often requires the coordinated efforts of an interprofessional team.

Another term often used is *children with special health care needs.* Children with IDD often have special health care needs, but this may not be true of all members of this population. For example, a child with Down syndrome may have special needs, but these special needs may not always concern the child's health at any given time.

As new terminology comes into use, it is important to identify and describe particular conditions (e.g., pervasive developmental disabilities and special needs child), so that nurses do not lose sight of the knowledge and skills needed to care for persons with IDD, regardless of the diagnosis. Although the terms used to describe IDD may overlap (e.g., *developmental disabilities* and *special health care needs* in the child with cerebral palsy), the definition of intellectual and developmental disabilities is used in federal legislation and must be understood by nurses.

History of Nursing in IDD

The history of nursing in IDD is unique. This section gives a short summary of the education of nurses and nursing care in this specialty.

Early education for nurses who specialized in the care of persons, of any age, with IDD occurred both in general nursing hospital schools and in asylums and institutions. Until the early 20th century, persons with IDD were diagnosed as having mental illness, and their care took place in settings where persons with all forms of mental illness were housed. It was not until after WWI, when a better understanding of mental illness occurred, that the care of persons with IDD was more specifically detailed. Terminology at this time included *idiot* and *imbecile.* In the early 1960s, President Kennedy brought needed attention to the living conditions of persons of all ages with IDD, then called *mental retardation.* New legislation was introduced and for the first time funding became available for this population. Large institutional settings remained the primary place of residence for persons of all ages with IDD until the late 1960s. It was the social norm to place newborns and children with known conditions resulting in IDD in institutions as soon as possible so as not to burden the families, either financially or through social stigma.

After public attention to the custodial and often inhumane care of persons with IDD in the early 1970s, radical changes took place. Many individuals with IDD were moved back to their homes and to newly formed community settings, such as group homes, semi-independent living arrangements (SILAs), and smaller congregate settings (e.g., 16 beds). The transition from institutional to community living varies state by state. Today, newborns with IDD are no longer placed in institutional settings. Most individuals with IDD live with their families in the community. Others live in small-group community settings; only the most severely affected individuals who require substantial medical care remain in larger developmental centers (Nehring, 1999).

Nursing care has also evolved throughout history. Early documentation about nursing care was written either by physicians or nurses who cared for both persons with IDD and mental illness. Specific literature on the nursing care of persons with IDD written by nurses first appeared with any frequency in the 1950s. At that time, nurses in institutional settings did little more than record vital signs and occasional patient weights and give medications. Public health nurses also provided care for children with IDD who remained at home. However, parents were often encouraged to enroll their children in institutions by the time they reached school age. The first national meeting for nurses specializing in the care of children with IDD was sponsored by the Children's Bureau in 1958 (Nehring, 1999).

In the 1960s, nursing care in the institution resembled the nursing care provided in hospitals. The role of the nurse expanded to include education and research. Advanced practice registered nurses were employed by some institutions and postbaccalaureate and graduate programs emerged to provide education designed especially for the care of children and adolescents with IDD. Interdisciplinary faculty (including nurses) at university-affiliated programs and facilities (UAPs or UAFs), established by President Kennedy in universities across the country, offered interdisciplinary education to future specialists in this field (including nurses), conducted research on topics related to mental retardation, and provided health and social services to individuals with IDD and their families.

Nurses began to write more prolifically about the care of children with IDD conditions; the increased numbers of articles and books; some of which are now considered classics, were especially useful for public health nurses. Developmental diagnostic clinics were established across the country to identify and refer children for developmental and health care when appropriate. Nursing consultants who specialized in this field were hired by the Children's Bureau; Division of Neurological Diseases and Stroke, U.S. Public Health Service; Mental Retardation Division, Department of Health, Education, and Welfare; Association of Retarded Children; and the United Cerebral Palsy Associations, Inc. National meetings were convened for these nursing specialists and the first standards of nursing practice for this specialty emerged in 1968, *The Guidelines for Nursing Standards in Residential Centers for the Mentally Retarded* (Haynes, 1968; Nehring, 1999).

The 1970s saw the first education legislation mandating that all children with IDD receive a free and appropriate public education from the ages of 3 through 21 years. Advanced practice roles for nurses in this specialty continued to expand, including roles in schools and early intervention programs for the infant from birth to three years of age. Publications and regular national and regional meetings continued to be held throughout this decade. Special courses in this area also began to appear in nursing programs across the country (Nehring, 1999).

The term *developmental disabilities* was first introduced during the Nixon presidency to describe conditions similar to those defined as mental retardation but that differed slightly. Interdisciplinary care was the norm in the 1980s, when all disciplines worked together with the individual with IDD and his or her family members in assessing and planning the care of the person with IDD in a variety of settings (Nehring, 1999). In 1980, the American Nurses Association published *School Nurses Working with Handicapped Children* (Igoe, Green, Heim, Licata, MacDonough, & McHugh, 1980). Later in the 1980s, two sets of standards of nursing practice for nurses specializing in this field emerged: *Standards of Nursing Practice in Mental Retardation/Developmental Disabilities* (Aggen & Moore, 1984) and *Standards for the Clinical Advanced Practice Registered Nurse in Developmental Disabilities/Handicapping Conditions* (Austin, Challela, Huber, Sciarillo, & Stade, 1987).

Emphasis on the adult with IDD emerged in the nursing literature in the 1990s. An examination of the individual with IDD across the lifespan was first highlighted in *A Life-Span Approach to Nursing Care for Individuals with Developmental Disabilities* (Roth & Morse, 1994). Nursing standards for this field were also revised: *Standards of Developmental Disabilities Nursing Practice* (Aggen, DeGennaro, Fox, Hahn, Logan, & VonFumetti, 1995) and *Statement on the Scope and Standards for the Nurse Who Specializes in Developmental Disabilities and/or Mental Retardation* (Nursing Division of the American Association on Mental Retardation and American Nurses Association, 1998). Other related standards of nursing practice in early intervention (ANA Consensus Committee, 1993), care of children and adolescents with special health and developmental needs (ANA Consensus Committee, 1994), and genetics (ISONG & ANA, 1998) were issued as well.

In the first years of the 21st century, a greater effort was made to provide educational materials for nursing students and nurses in practice who care for persons of all ages with IDD. Both the Nursing Division of the American Association on Mental Retardation and the Developmental Disabilities Nurses Association have been developing separate, but complementary, projects to create a core curriculum for nurses and other health professionals (Nehring, 2005) and Internet materials, respectively.

This specialty field of nursing has changed greatly from its early years. As the healthcare system continues to evolve, so will the nursing care of persons of all ages with IDD. Such care continues to occur in a variety of settings and at both the professional registered nurse and advanced practice registered nurse levels. Continued publication and research into such nursing care are needed, as are additional didactic and clinical content materials for nursing students.

Professional Nursing's Scope and Standards of IDD Nursing Practice

For more than a decade, nurse members of the American Association on Intellectual and Developmental Disabilities (AAIDD) have deemed it important that there be a scope and standards of practice for this specialty. This document serves as the contemporary template for the practice of nursing in IDD, and the standards of practice portion of this document serves as a description of the practice of nurses who specialize in this field.

Description of the Scope of IDD Nursing Practice

The scope of practice statement describes the *who, what, where, when, why,* and *how* of nursing practice. Each of these questions must be answered to provide a complete picture of the dynamic and complex practice of IDD nursing and its evolving boundaries and membership. The full spectrum of the nurse's role in this specialty is described for both the general and advanced practice registered nurse. The depth and breadth with which individual registered nurses engage in the total scope of nursing practice for this specialty depend on each nurse's education, experience, role, and the population served.

Development and Function of IDD Nursing Standards

The Standards of Professional Nursing Practice in IDD Nursing are authoritative statements of the duties that all registered nurses in this specialty are expected to perform competently. The standards published herein may serve as evidence of the standard of care for this specialty, with the understanding that application of the standards depends on context. The standards are subject to change with the dynamics of this nursing specialty, as new patterns of professional practice are developed and accepted by the nursing profession and the public. In addition, specific conditions and clinical circumstances may also affect the application of these standards at a given time, such as during a natural disaster. The standards are subject to formal, periodic review and revision.

The Function of Competencies in IDD Nursing Standards

The competencies that accompany each standard may be evidence of compliance with the corresponding standard. The list of competencies is not exhaustive. Whether a particular standard or competency applies depends on the circumstances.

The Nursing Process in IDD Nursing

The *nursing process* is often conceptualized as the integration of singular actions of assessment, diagnosis, and identification of outcomes, planning, implementation, and finally, evaluation. The nursing process in practice is not linear, as often conceptualized, with a single feedback loop from evaluation to assessment. Rather, it relies heavily on bidirectional feedback loops from each component, as illustrated in Figure 1. There is no deviation in this process for nurses specializing in IDD.

The Standards of Practice for IDD Nurses coincide with the steps of the nursing process, to represent the directive nature of the standards as the IDD professional nurse completes each component of the nursing process. Similarly, the Standards of Professional Performance for IDD Nurses relate to how the IDD professional nurse adheres to the Standards of Practice for IDD Nurses, completes the nursing process, and addresses other nursing practice issues and concerns (ANA, 2010a). Five tenets characterize contemporary nursing practice, and these are described here for the IDD nurse.

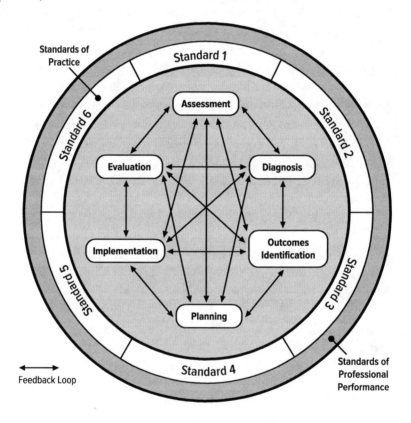

FIGURE 1. The Nursing Process and Standards of Professional Nursing Practice (ANA, 2010a)

Tenets Characteristic of IDD Nursing Practice

1. IDD nursing practice is individualized.

IDD nursing practice respects diversity and is individualized to meet the unique needs of the healthcare consumer with IDD or situation. The *healthcare consumer with IDD* is defined to be the patient, person, client, family/legal guardians, group, community, or population with IDD who is the focus of attention and to whom the IDD registered nurse is providing services as sanctioned by the state regulatory bodies.

2. IDD nurses coordinate care by establishing partnerships.

The IDD registered nurse establishes partnerships with persons with IDD, families/legal guardians, support systems, and other providers, and uses in-person and electronic communications to reach a shared goal of delivering health care. *Health care* is defined as the attempt "to address the health needs of the patient and the public" (ANA, 2001, p.10). Collaborative interprofessional team planning is based on recognition of each discipline's value and contributions, mutual trust, respect, open discussion, and shared decision-making.

3. Caring is central to the practice of the IDD registered nurse.

IDD professional nursing promotes healing and health in a way that builds a relationship between the IDD nurse and the healthcare consumer with IDD (Watson, 1999, 2008). "Caring is a conscious judgment that manifests itself in concrete acts, interpersonally, verbally, and nonverbally" (Gallagher-Lepak & Kubsch, 2009, p. 171). While caring for healthcare consumers with IDD, families/legal guardians, and populations is the key focus of IDD nursing, the IDD nurse additionally promotes self-care as well as care of the environment and society (Hagerty, Lynch-Sauer, Patusky, & Bouwseman, 1993).

4. IDD registered nurses use the nursing process to plan and provide individualized care to their healthcare consumers with IDD.

IDD nurses use theoretical and evidence-based knowledge of human experiences and responses to collaborate with healthcare consumers with IDD to assess, diagnose, identify outcomes, plan, implement, and evaluate care. IDD nursing interventions are intended to produce beneficial effects, contribute to quality outcomes, and—above all—do no harm. IDD nurses evaluate the effectiveness of their care in relation to identified outcomes and use evidence-based practice to improve care (ANA, 2010a). Critical thinking underlies each step of the nursing process, problem-solving, and decision-making. The nursing process is cyclical and dynamic, interpersonal and collaborative, and universally applicable.

5. A strong link exists between the professional work environment and the IDD registered nurse's ability to provide quality health care and achieve optimal outcomes.

IDD professional nurses have an ethical obligation to maintain and improve healthcare practice environments conducive to the provision of quality health care (ANA, 2010b). Extensive studies have demonstrated the relationship between effective nursing practice and the presence of a healthy work environment (e.g., Aiken, Clarke, Sloane, Lake, & Cheney, 2008; Kelly, McHugh, & Aiken, 2011; Papastavrou et al., 2011). Mounting evidence demonstrates that negative, demoralizing, and unsafe conditions in the workplace (unhealthy work environments) contribute to medical errors, ineffective delivery of care, and conflict and stress among health professionals. IDD nurses are similarly affected.

Healthy Work Environments for IDD Nursing Practice

ANA supports the following models of healthy work environment design. These concepts apply to the healthy work environments of IDD nursing practice as well.

American Association of Critical Care Nurses

The American Association of Critical Care Nurses has identified six standards for establishing and maintaining healthy work environments (AACN, 2005):

- *Skilled Communication* Nurses must be as proficient in communication skills as they are in clinical skills.

- *True Collaboration* Nurses must be relentless in pursuing and fostering a sense of team and partnership across all disciplines.

- *Effective Decision-Making* Nurses are seen as valued and committed partners in making policy, directing and evaluating clinical care, and leading organizational operations.

- *Appropriate Staffing* Staffing must ensure the effective match between healthcare consumer needs and nurse competencies.

- *Meaningful Recognition* Nurses must be recognized and must recognize others for the value each brings to the work of the organization.

- *Authentic Leadership* Nurse leaders must fully embrace the imperative of a healthy work environment, authentically live it, and engage others in achieving it.

Magnet Recognition Program®

The Magnet Recognition Program® addresses the professional work environment, requiring that Magnet®-designated facilities adhere to the following model components [American Nurses Credentialing Center (ANCC), 2008]:

- *Transformational Leadership* The transformational leader leads people where they need to be in order to meet the demands of the future.

- *Structural Empowerment* Structures and processes developed by influential leadership provide an innovative practice environment in which strong professional practice flourishes and the mission, vision, and values come to life to achieve the outcomes believed to be important for the organization.

- *Exemplary Professional Practice* This demonstrates what professional nursing practice can achieve.

- *New Knowledge, Innovation, and Improvements* Organizations have an ethical and professional responsibility to contribute to healthcare delivery, the organization, and the profession.

- *Empirical Quality Results* Organizations are in a unique position to become pioneers of the future and to demonstrate solutions to numerous problems inherent in today's healthcare systems. Beyond the "what" and "how," organizations must ask themselves what difference these efforts have made.

Institute of Medicine

The Institute of Medicine has also reported that safety and quality problems occur when dedicated health professionals work in systems that neither support them nor prepare them to achieve optimal patient care outcomes (IOM, 2004). Such rapid changes as reimbursement modification and cost-containment efforts, new healthcare technologies, and changes in the healthcare workforce have influenced the work and work environment of nurses. Accordingly, concentration on key aspects of the work environment of IDD nursing practice—people, physical surroundings, and tools—can enhance healthcare working conditions and improve patient safety. These include:

- Transformational leadership and evidence-based management

- Maximizing workforce capability

- Creating and sustaining a culture of safety and research

- Workspace design and redesign to prevent and mitigate errors

- Effective use of telecommunications and biomedical device interoperability

Model of Professional Nursing Practice Regulation

In 2006, the Model of Professional Nursing Practice Regulation (see Figure 2) emerged from ANA work and informed the discussions of specialty nursing and advanced practice registered nurse practice. This Model of

Professional Nursing Practice Regulation applies equally to IDD specialty nursing practice.

The lowest level in the model represents the responsibility of the IDD professional and specialty nursing organizations to their members and the public to define the scope and standards of practice for IDD nursing.

The next level up the pyramid represents the regulation provided by the nurse practice acts, rules, and regulations in the pertinent licensing jurisdictions. Institutional policies and procedures provide further considerations in the regulation of nursing practice for the IDD registered nurse and IDD advanced practice registered nurse.

Note that the highest level is that of self-determination by the IDD nurse, after consideration of all the other levels of input about professional

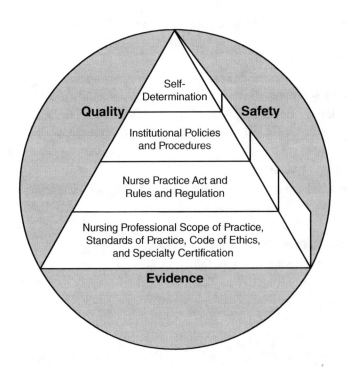

FIGURE 2. Model of Professional Nursing Practice Regulation
(Styles, Schumann, Bickford, & White, 2008)

nursing practice regulation. The outcome is safe, quality, and evidence-based practice.

Standards of Professional Nursing Practice in IDD

The Standards of Professional Nursing Practice in IDD are comprised of the Standards of Practice in IDD and the Standards of Professional Performance in IDD.

Standards of Practice in IDD Nursing

The Standards of Practice in IDD Nursing describe a competent level of IDD nursing care as demonstrated by the critical thinking model known as the nursing process. The nursing process includes the components of assessment, diagnosis, outcomes identification, planning, implementation, and evaluation. Accordingly, the nursing process encompasses significant actions taken by IDD registered nurses and forms the foundation of the nurse's decision-making.

STANDARD 1. ASSESSMENT

The registered nurse who specializes in IDD collects comprehensive data pertinent to the healthcare consumer's health and/or the situation.

STANDARD 2. DIAGNOSIS

The registered nurse who specializes in IDD analyzes the assessment data to determine the diagnoses or the issues.

STANDARD 3. OUTCOMES IDENTIFICATION

The registered nurse who specializes in IDD identifies expected outcomes for a plan individualized to the healthcare consumer with IDD or the situation.

STANDARD 4. PLANNING

The registered nurse who specializes in IDD develops a plan that prescribes strategies and alternatives to attain expected outcomes.

STANDARD 5. IMPLEMENTATION

The registered nurse who specializes in IDD implements the identified plan.

STANDARD 5A. COORDINATION OF CARE

The registered nurse who specializes in IDD coordinates care delivery.

STANDARD 5B. HEALTH TEACHING AND HEALTH PROMOTION

The registered nurse who specializes in IDD employs strategies to promote health and a safe environment.

STANDARD 5C. CONSULTATION

The advanced practice registered nurse who specializes in IDD provides consultation to influence the identified plan, enhance the abilities of others, and effect change.

STANDARD 5D. PRESCRIPTIVE AUTHORITY AND TREATMENT

The advanced practice registered nurse who specializes in IDD uses prescriptive authority, procedures, referrals, treatments, and therapies in accordance with state and federal laws and regulations.

STANDARD 6. EVALUATION

The registered nurse who specializes in IDD evaluates progress toward attainment of outcomes.

Standards of Professional Performance in IDD Nursing

The Standards of Professional Performance in IDD Nursing describe a competent level of behavior in the professional role, including activities related to ethics, education, evidence-based practice and research, quality of practice, communication, leadership, collaboration, professional practice evaluation, resource utilization, and environmental health. All IDD registered nurses are expected to engage in professional role activities, including leadership, appropriate to their education and position. IDD registered nurses are accountable for their professional actions to themselves, their healthcare consumers with IDD, their peers, and ultimately to society.

STANDARD 7. ETHICS

The registered nurse who specializes in IDD practices ethically.

STANDARD 8. EDUCATION

The registered nurse who specializes in IDD attains knowledge and competence that reflect current nursing practice.

STANDARD 9. EVIDENCE-BASED PRACTICE AND RESEARCH

The registered nurse who specializes in IDD integrates evidence and research findings into practice.

STANDARD 10. QUALITY OF PRACTICE

The registered nurse who specializes in IDD contributes to quality nursing practice.

STANDARD 11. COMMUNICATION

The registered nurse who specializes in IDD communicates effectively in a variety of formats in all areas of practice.

STANDARD 12. LEADERSHIP

The registered nurse who specializes in IDD demonstrates leadership in the professional practice setting and the profession.

STANDARD 13. COLLABORATION

The registered nurse who specializes in IDD collaborates with the healthcare consumer with IDD, family/legal guardians, and others in the conduct of nursing practice.

STANDARD 14. PROFESSIONAL PRACTICE EVALUATION

The registered nurse who specializes in IDD evaluates her or his own nursing practice in relation to professional practice standards and guidelines, relevant statutes, rules, and regulations.

STANDARD 15. RESOURCE UTILIZATION
The registered nurse who specializes in IDD utilizes appropriate resources to plan and provide nursing services that are safe, effective, and financially responsible to healthcare consumers with IDD.

STANDARD 16. ENVIRONMENTAL HEALTH
The registered nurse who specializes in IDD practices in an environmentally safe and healthy manner.

Professional Competence in IDD Nursing Practice

The public has a right to expect IDD registered nurses to demonstrate professional competence throughout their careers. The IDD registered nurse is individually responsible and accountable for maintaining professional competence. It is the nursing profession's responsibility to shape and guide any process for assuring nurse competence. Regulatory agencies define minimal standards of competence to protect the public. The employer is responsible and accountable to provide a practice environment conducive to competent practice. Assurance of competence is the shared responsibility of the profession, individual nurses, professional organizations, credentialing entities, regulatory agencies, employers, and other key stakeholders (ANA, 2008).

ANA believes that in the practice of nursing, competence can be defined, measured, and evaluated. No single evaluation method or tool can guarantee competence. Competence is situational and dynamic; it is both an outcome and an ongoing process. Context determines what competencies are necessary. Nurses working in specialty areas, such as with individuals with IDD, are responsible for general nursing competence as well as the skills and knowledge required for the specific population of concern. Standards for any specialty must be dynamic and reflective of the current state of knowledge and evidence-based practice. Development of standards of competence was recommended by the Institute of Medicine to improve healthcare education and enhance the ability of healthcare providers to care for very complex patients (IOM, 2001, 2003), a term that describes many individuals with IDD.

Definitions and Concepts Related to Competence in IDD Nursing

The National Council of State Boards of Nursing defined *competence* as "the application of knowledge and the interpersonal, decision-making, and psycho-motor skills expected for the practice role, within the context of public health" (NCSBN, 2005, p. 81). *Competence* has also been defined as the description of a behavior or act, while *competency* has been defined as the underlying behavior that leads to the competent performance (McMullan et al., 2003). Competence is composed of varied attributes, including judgment, critical thinking skills, and physical/behavioral skills. Competence is job related and situation related, and represents qualities that yield effective performance on the job. Competence is the capacity and potential to perform in a given set-ting (Cowan, Norman, & Coopamah, 2007). Competence is the application and demonstration of skills, knowledge, and judgment (Scott Tilley, 2008). Benner (1984) proposed a developmental model of competence with stages from novice to expert, which posits that competence is also dependent on length of experience. Because nursing education by and large lacks content and experience in care of individuals with IDD, nurses must learn on the job or through continuing education.

Competence and Competency in IDD Nursing Practice

A variety of intrinsic and extrinsic factors influence competence in actual day-to-day nursing practice. Quality care results from competence. Environmental factors may be supportive of competency or present challenges. For example, performing a physical exam on a cooperative patient may be a basic skill, but performing a physical exam on an individual with autism, a sensory disorder, and a communication disorder may require a different set of knowledge, dif-fering expertise, and unusual patience.

There is little empirical data to inform care of individuals with IDD and to guide competence in nursing practice with this population. The majority of nurses entering into practice have little or no experience with children or adults with IDD, and many believe they will never encounter such persons in practice. However, as more individuals with IDD leave institutions and live in the community, nurses in all settings, including school nurses, will find them-selves involved in services for the IDD population.

Lazarus and Lee (2006) studied healthcare consumers' identification of factors they believed influenced nursing competence. Education, number of patients, hours worked, education in procedures, salary, involvement in professional activities, attitude, and work conditions were among the factors listed. Excessive work hours and poor work conditions translated to poor quality of care. Behaviors such as lack of courtesy and caring, poor communication skills, discomfort with performing technical skills, and knowledge deficits negatively influenced competence (Lazarus & Lee, 2006). Behaviors such as these put all patients at risk, and are particularly risky for individuals with intellectual and developmental disability due to their vulnerabilities.

The registered nurse who specializes in IDD systematically enhances the quality and effectiveness of nursing practice by performing care according to quality standards and by meeting both generalist and specialist nursing competencies. Lifelong learning is a commitment to quality, requiring nurses to constantly reappraise their own practice and seek to upgrade knowledge and skills (American Nurses Association & the Nursing Division of the American Association on Mental Retardation, 2004).

Evaluating Competence in IDD Nurses

Competence in nursing practice must be evaluated by the individual nurse (self assessment), nurse peers, and nurses in the roles of supervisor, coach, mentor, or preceptor. In addition, other aspects of nursing performance may be evaluated by professional colleagues and patients.

Competence can be evaluated by using tools that capture objective and subjective data about the individual's knowledge base and actual performance and are appropriate for the specific situation and the desired outcome of the competence evaluation. . . . However, no single evaluation tool or method can guarantee competence. (ANA, 2008, p. 6)

Bachelor's- and associate-level programs prepare nurses to meet general nursing competencies and to pass the NCLEX licensing exams upon graduation. Graduation from an accredited program and successful completion of the licensing exam represent to the public, consumers, and employers that the registered nurse is capable of general, competent, and safe nursing care. The IOM (IOM, 2010) recommends that all graduating RNs complete a nurse internship before entering into independent practice. Currently, this occurs mostly in the hospital setting, but nurse internships in community agencies serving individuals with IDD would allow novice registered nurses to hone the basic skills they developed in training and apply them to the needs of the IDD population.

Continuing education has traditionally been the primary method of evaluating competence for practicing registered nurses, as well as many advanced practice registered nurses (APRNs). Nursing organizations [such as the Developmental Disabilities Nursing Association (DDNA)] offer certification of registered nurses (separate from APRN certification) as one method of evaluating competence of professional nurses working in specialized settings. The registered nurse who specializes in IDD evaluates her or his own nursing practice in relation to professional practice standards and evidence-based guidelines, and relevant statutes, rules, and regulations, identifying strengths and areas in need of further development. As part of the self-evaluation of practice, the registered nurse solicits feedback from healthcare consumers, family members/legal guardians, colleagues, and others, including direct care support professionals. Use of practice portfolios places the responsibility of maintaining competence on the individual nurse, and can document experience in subspecialties (such as care of individuals with IDD), involvement in quality assurance efforts, and participation in professional interdisciplinary and nursing specialty organizations, as well as competencies not evaluated by other methods. The IDD nurse must also evaluate nursing care delegated to other professionals, direct care support professionals, unlicensed assistive personnel, or the family/legal guardians and document the effect of delegation on health outcomes (American Nurses Association & Nursing Division of the American Association on Mental Retardation, 2004).

Professional Registered IDD Nurses Today

Statistical Snapshot

There are approximately 2.6 million licensed registered nurses employed in the United States (Bureau of Labor Statistics, May 2011), about 9% of whom are APRNs. Other positions held by nurses include administrative, educational, and academic/research posts. The number of nurses identifying themselves as IDD nurses is unknown. The only national certification for registered nurses specifically addressing individuals with IDD is the Developmental Disabilities Nurses Association (DDNA), which claims about 1,300 members, including LPNs, associate's-degree registered nurses, and baccalaureate-prepared registered nurses, as well as APRNs and doctorally prepared nurses. Interdisciplinary organizations such as the American Association on Intellectual and Developmental Disabilities (AAIDD) and the International Association for the Scientific Study of Intellectual Disability (IASSID) count nurses among their membership. Nurses practicing in other specialties such as orthopedics, rehabilitation, psychiatric nursing, neurology/neurosurgery, and pediatric nursing frequently encounter children and adults with IDD. In fact, nurses working in any inpatient or outpatient setting are likely to encounter people with IDD, since 75% of the population of almost 600,000 individuals with IDD live in community settings (Braddock, Hemp, Rizzolo, Haffer, Tanis, & Wu, 2011).

Licensure and Education of IDD Registered Nurses

The IDD registered nurse is licensed and authorized by a state, commonwealth, or territory to practice nursing. Licensure of the healthcare professions is established by each jurisdiction to protect the public safety and authorize the practice of the profession. Because of this, the licensure requirements for RNs and advanced practice nursing vary widely.

Although most professional nursing organizations, such as ANA, emphasize that bachelor's preparation in nursing is the entry into practice, many community colleges and private educational institutions still offer the associate's degree for registered nurses, particularly when there are local or national shortages of registered nurses. Associate's-degree graduates take the same national licensing exam (NCLEX) as baccalaureate graduates. Accredited baccalaureate (BSN) and associate's-degree (AD) programs differ somewhat, but all must address the basic competencies needed for the NCLEX exam. Entry-level registered nurses are prepared as generalists, and often specialize following graduation and licensure. More programs now exist that offer a pathway from AD to BSN, and above (Kearney, 2009).

Registered nurses may pursue advanced academic studies to prepare for specialization in practice. Educational requirements vary by specialty and educational program. New models for educational preparation are evolving in response to the changing healthcare, education, and regulatory practice environments.

Advanced practice registered nurses (APRNs) include clinical nurse specialists (CNS), certified nurse practitioners (CNP), certified nurse midwives (CNM), and certified registered nurse anesthetists (CRNA). APRNs are registered as such, in addition to their registered nurse licensure, with the state board of nursing in the state where they reside. However, current regulation of APRNs varies widely across the states. The APRN Joint Dialogue Group (2008) proposed a model of practice and state regulation for advanced practice registered nurses which, when adopted by all states and specialty nursing organizations, will facilitate assessment of competence. Graduate-prepared nurses who are not involved in direct patient care (such as those in administration, informatics, public health, or education) will not be subject to the *Consensus Model for APRN Regulation: Licensure, Accreditation, Certification & Education* (APRN Joint Dialogue Group, 2008).

Nurses with a master's degree may continue their education toward the Doctor of Philosophy (PhD) degree or the Doctor of Nursing Practice (DNP) degree. The PhD graduate focuses on research and theory generation, as well as academic education. The DNP graduate focuses on clinical practice, quality assurance, and clinical outcome evaluation, as well as clinical education in academic and other settings.

In the United States, the student in the basic nursing education program leading to licensure as a registered nurse is not prepared to specialize in IDD. Continuing education programs and progressive work experience with those who have intellectual and developmental disabilities enhance the IDD nurse's knowledge, skills, and abilities. At the graduate level, a few programs across the country do offer specialization in IDD, and these programs are funded by the Maternal and Child Health Bureau. A listing of these programs can be found on the Maternal and Child Health Bureau web site (http://www.mchb.hrsa.gov/training/; from the home page, indicate "nursing" in the field asking for discipline).

Roots of Professional IDD Nursing

As with the discipline of nursing in general, the nursing specialty of IDD uses the nursing process to assess and identify health problems, determine desired outcomes, plan and implement, and evaluate the effectiveness of interventions. IDD nursing has evolved into a profession with a distinct body of knowledge, university-based education, and specialized practice. (For a complete discussion of the history of IDD nursing, see Nehring, 1999.) Nursing care in this specialty is defined by the standards of nursing practice and professional performance for nurses who specialize in IDD, as well as the scope and standards of care for professional nurses (ANA, 2010a). The practice of APRNs who specialize in caring for individuals with IDD must also be congruent with their chosen role (e.g., NP, CNS, CRNA, CNM) as well as their population focus (adult/geriatric, family, neonatal, pediatric, women's health, and psychiatric/mental health) (APRN Joint Dialogue Group, 2008 & National Council of State Boards of Nursing APRN Advisory Committee, 2008; American Nurses Association & Nursing Division of the American Association on Mental Retardation, 2004).

IDD Nursing Research and Evidence-Based Practice

Dorothea Dix is thought to be the first leader in IDD nursing. Although Dix was not a nurse, she is viewed by many as being instrumental in the development of IDD, public health, and mental health nursing (Nehring, 1999). Using her careful observations of the living conditions of individuals with IDD, Dix made many appeals for more hygienic buildings for individuals with IDD and mental illness, and some of her efforts met with success (Dix, 1847). For example, she spoke to the Massachusetts legislature in 1843 about the conditions of jails, asylums, and almshouses in Massachusetts (Dix, 1976). Consistent with Florence Nightingale's call for nurses to use their observations to bring about change (Nightingale, 1859), Dix used her observations to inform and influence legislators to improve the living conditions of individuals with IDD (Nehring, 1999).

In the 1960s, nurses began conducting and publishing their research about individuals with IDD. These early nurse researchers relied on models, research findings, and/or research methods from the fields of education, medicine, physical therapy, cognitive and developmental psychology, psychiatry, public health, speech therapy, and sociology. Miller (1979) described a program that was implemented from 1962 through 1964 to teach personnel in the Central Wisconsin Colony and Training School to provide speech and physical therapy to residents. Pat McNelly (1966) conducted a study that "was a precursor to development of the transdisciplinary model of care delivery" (Nehring, 1999, p. 79). A cross-disciplinary project, the Mimosa Project, was funded to teach adolescent girls with IDD daily living skills (Devine, 1983). Barclay, Goulet, Holtgrewe, and Sharp (1962) examined parents' evaluations of the clinic services provided to their children with IDD. By 1970, many studies related to IDD had been or were being carried out by nurses, and graduate students in nursing programs were focusing their dissertation research on IDD. Between 1970 and 2000, more than 100 nursing dissertations related to IDD were completed (Nehring, 1999).

Nurses contribute to research and scholarly work related to IDD across the lifespan. Two nurses who are well recognized for their work in developmental disabilities focused their work on infants and children with or at risk for IDD. Una H. Haynes, a committed nurse who made many contributions to the field of developmental disabilities, was on the national staff team of the United Cerebral Palsy Associations, Inc., and is credited with developing the transdisciplinary approach to early intervention for infants with developmental disabilities (Haynes, 1974). Kathryn Barnard began her work with children with IDD (Barnard, 1966, 1968), developed the Nursing Child Assessment Satellite Training (NCAST) Scales that have been widely used to assess parent–infant interactions (Sumner & Spietz, 1994), and has been an advocate for prevention in nursing and mental health. She serves as director of the Center on Infant Mental Health and Development at the University of Washington.

Just as nursing research has evolved and developed across the profession, nursing research in IDD has evolved and continues its development, including an emphasis on evidence-based practice. Quantitative, qualitative, and mixed-methods studies are conducted across the lifespan using nursing and non-nursing theories. Nurses working in the field of IDD have long recognized the importance of interprofessional collaboration in practice. Likewise, interprofessional collaboration is essential for many nursing research activities and the identification and implementation of evidence-based practice related to IDD.

Nurse researchers have focused their research on specific conditions that result in or are associated with IDD, roles and responsibilities of nurses working in this field, families/legal guardians and family-centered care, and education of nurses and others about IDD. Nehring (1999) called for research that (a) evaluates programs and services provided to individuals with IDD;

(b) examines adult health care, adult development, and the educational needs of caregivers across the lifespan of individuals with IDD; (c) explores issues related to genetics; and (d) explores the perspectives of individuals with IDD and their families/legal guardians that need to be addressed by nurses. Although these areas continue to draw the attention of nurse researchers, new challenges related to the complexities of health care and demands for healthcare reform also require attention. Nurse researchers should examine nursing practice in IDD to demonstrate that staffing is adequate to ensure quality care for individuals with IDD and their families/legal guardians. Consistent with the call for continual evaluation of nursing practice, as stated in *Nursing's Social Policy Statement* (ANA, 2010b), ongoing evaluation of patient outcomes and learning needs of nurses working with individuals with IDD and their families/legal guardians, and dissemination of information to address these outcomes and needs, are critical.

IDD Specialty Practice in Nursing

All nurses will care for an individual with IDD sometime in their career. Each person with IDD is a person first, just like everyone else, and each person's healthcare needs are unique to that individual. It is important that nurses recognize that a person with IDD (a) is not sick based on the diagnosis of a IDD, (b) does not necessarily have all of the secondary conditions identified as common to the diagnosis (e.g., a person with spina bifida does not always have hydrocephaly), and (c) experiences many of the same life events (e.g., graduation, first job, etc.) and has the same feelings that all of us do. It is important that diagnostic overshadowing (attributing a health problem to the person's diagnosis of IDD; e.g., an adolescent with Down syndrome who is depressed because he broke up with his girlfriend is thought to be depressed because he has Down syndrome) does not occur. In most prelicensure nursing programs, the attention focused on care of persons with IDD is small, but nurses practicing as registered nurses must be able to provide holistic care to this population. Many books, articles, videos, and Internet sites are available to assist in this learning. The registered nurse may also want to consult with a nurse specialist in this field.

The registered nurse who specializes in IDD provides care to individuals, families/legal guardians, and groups in a wide range of care settings, based on an understanding of the concepts and strategies of nursing practice in this area. The registered nurse participates in implementation of individual and family/legal guardians' assessment and in the planning, implementation, and evaluation of their health and health services. If an APRN is not available, the registered nurse may serve as a case manager as part of an interprofessional team for healthcare consumers with IDD who have less complex needs. The registered nurse collaborates and consults with the APRN in IDD as a resource. If no APRN is available in the practice setting, one may be able to find an APRN who can serve as a consultant through DDNA, the Health and Wellness Action Group of the AAIDD, or University Centers of Excellence in Developmental Disabilities (UCEDDs, formerly UAPs or UAFs).

Advanced Practice IDD Registered Nurse Roles

The majority of APRNs will care for some persons with IDD during their careers. The nurse practitioner may encounter the pregnant woman with an IDD, the birth of a child with an IDD, the diagnosis of IDD in a child, the care of a child with IDD throughout childhood and adolescence to the transition to adulthood and adult health care, adult health services, psychiatric-mental health services, and finally, older adult services. The nurse practitioner may carry out these services in the clinic, hospital, school, home, or residential setting. The clinical nurse specialist, in any area of specialty, may encounter the person with IDD in the hospital or clinic setting. The nurse midwife will most likely be involved, at some point, in the birth of a child with IDD or care for a woman with IDD who is having a baby. The nurse anesthetist may also care for an individual with IDD who is undergoing surgery. As in prelicensure nursing education, graduate nursing programs give little attention to the health care needs of persons, of any age, with IDD, unless the student chooses to specialize in this field. All nurses, regardless of educational preparation, must be prepared for the unique health care needs of persons with IDD and always include the individual's family/legal guardians and additional support persons, if applicable, in all discussions of care. As stated earlier, many resources are available to nurses to enhance their knowledge and skills in this area, including consultation with master's and doctorally prepared nurse specialists in this field.

Specifically, the master's or doctorally prepared nurse who specializes in IDD is an APRN or specialist, who has the authority to perform all of the functions of the registered nurse with an independent and conceptually sophisticated focus. The master's-prepared nurse in this specialty may practice in a clinical role, or may work with and for healthcare consumers with IDD through a higher level of preparation in nursing administration, nursing education, public health nursing, or informatics. Certification is obtained for the specific role and age group (e.g., pediatric nurse practitioner).

In addition, the APRN and master's-prepared nurse possesses:

- Substantial experience with individuals with IDD, their families/legal guardians, and community resources;

- Skill in the formulation and implementation of social policy and legislation affecting persons with IDD;

- The ability to plan, implement, and evaluate programs designed to serve individuals with IDD and their families/legal guardians; and

- The ability to conduct research.

These skills are based upon knowledge of specific intellectual and developmental disabilities, including their epidemiology and demographics. The APRN understands the use of adaptive technology for persons with IDD, as well as the impact of social, psychological, educational, cultural, and religious values on individuals, their families/legal guardians, and communities. Knowledge about cost containment, legislation, and policy planning enables the APRN to provide preventive, habilitative, supportive, and restorative care to healthcare consumers with IDD across the lifespan in a wide variety of settings. Case management, or care/service coordination, is also an important role (American Nurses Association & Nursing Division of the American Association on Mental Retardation, 2004).

The doctorally prepared nurse in this specialty may function in a clinical, educational, administrative, consulting, or research role. Nurses prepared at the Doctor of Philosophy (PhD) level focus on research, theory generation, and academic nursing education. More recently, the Doctor of Nursing Practice (DNP) degree has been established as a clinical doctorate in nursing. DNP-prepared APRNs working with individuals with IDD may be involved in clinical education about the population, evaluation of health care outcomes, or programmatic quality assurance.

Advanced Practice Registered Nurse is a regulatory title and includes the four roles listed earlier. The core competencies for education and the scope of practice are defined by the professional associations. State law and regulation further define criteria for licensure for the designated scopes of practice. The need to ensure healthcare consumer safety and access to APRNs, by aligning education, accreditation, licensure, and certification, is shown in *Consensus Model for APRN Regulation: Licensure, Accreditation, Certification & Education* (APRN Joint Dialogue Group, 2008). Organizations for each practice role have also established standards and competencies.

IDD Nurses in Advocacy and Society

Advocacy and a commitment to community inclusion are key characteristics of nurses working on behalf of people with IDD and their families/legal guardians. From advocacy with legislatures at the state and national levels, to individual advocacy supporting choice and self-determination for the individual with IDD, nurses in the specialty are passionate about the population and about achieving social justice for them. Assisting individuals with IDD to transition from an institutional setting into a less restrictive setting, such as their own home or a supervised apartment; to obtain quality health care; identifying and responding to allegations of abuse; and aiding in healthcare decision-making by supporting the individual or identifying a surrogate are all crucial areas for advocacy intervention.

Though there are many challenges in this field, such as communication difficulties, multiple comorbid conditions, public ignorance, and societal prejudice, there are also many rewards. Learning about and working with this population, for whom significant health disparities have only recently been identified, can enlighten and add meaning to nursing practice and personal life. Nurses learn to appreciate individuals' strengths and assist the individuals to cope and function in spite of their limitations (American Nurses Association & Nursing Division of the American Association on Mental Retardation, 2004).

Progression of IDD Nursing Education

ANA's long-held position is that the baccalaureate degree is the entry degree into nursing. Nevertheless, nursing's educational track to professional and career growth is not linear, and though there is an explicit progression of educational degrees, there is flexibility in how the progression is achieved. Educational bodies are establishing entry-into-practice master's programs, associate's-degree to baccalaureate- or master's-degree programs, and (most notably) second-degree baccalaureate programs.

As previously stated, nurses at all levels of education will, at some point in their careers, interact with healthcare consumers with IDD. The student enrolled in any educational program at any level may request to care for individuals of any age with IDD. It is important that students and nurses have exposure to this important population and that they are instructed in the knowledge, skills, and attitudes to appropriately and professionally provide care.

IOM Influences on the Quality and Environment of IDD Nursing Practice

The Institute of Medicine (IOM), a branch of the National Academies of Sciences, commissions reports on topics related to health care and healthcare services. The IOM does not necessarily represent nursing, but does involve nurses in its work. Three reports related to healthcare quality and safety have been released since 1999. The report titled, *To Err Is Human: Building a Safer Health System* (IOM, 1999) pointed out that faulty systems, rather than individuals, contributed significantly to the harm that was done to healthcare consumers. A second report, *Crossing the Quality Chasm: A New Health System for the 21st Century* (IOM, 2001), called for redesign of the entire health system to improve patient safety and quality outcomes and help retain health professionals who felt that their contributions were helping to improve patient care. The third report, *Keeping Patients Safe: Transforming the Work Environment of Nurses* (IOM, 2004), proposed changes in components of the workplace of nurses that would lead to better outcomes for patients and nurses. An analysis of the effects of nurse practice environments on nurse and patient outcomes by Aiken, Clarke, Sloane, Lake, and Cheney (2008) showed that patients in hospitals with a better practice environment fared far better than patients in hospitals with poor practice environments. These IOM reports, and the study by Aiken et al., have implications for IDD nursing. The work environment of nurses in IDD must allow nurses to meet their social responsibility for the healthcare safety of individuals with IDD.

An IOM report prepared by the Committee of the Robert Wood Johnson Foundation Initiative on the Future of Nursing at the IOM extended the focus on high-quality, safe, effective, evidence-based, and patient-centered care to a focus on the critical role of nursing and the association between the future of nursing and the future of the healthcare system (IOM, 2010). This report calls for (a) elimination of barriers that prevent nurses from practicing to the full extent of their education and training; (b) an improved education system that facilitates nurses' achievement of higher levels of education and training to ensure that nurses are providing safe, quality, patient-centered care; (c) redesign of the healthcare system in collaboration with other health professionals; and (d) improved data collection, data management infrastructure, and workforce planning. The practice of nurses varies from state to state depending on the regulations of each state. Nurses providing care to individuals with IDD should practice at the level to which they are prepared to practice and should be responsible for their own personal and professional growth. This includes developing leadership skills, mentoring others, and developing partnerships within and outside their healthcare environment. Careful collection and analysis of data on the healthcare professionals and nonprofessionals providing services to individuals with IDD are critical to assuring that a qualified healthcare workforce meets the needs of individuals with IDD.

The IOM has produced two specific documents related to individuals with IDD: *Disability in America: Toward a National Agenda for Prevention* (Pope & Tarlov, 1991) and *The Future of Disability in America* (Committee on Disability in America, Field, & Jette, 2007). The authors of the first document (Pope & Tarlov, 1991) discussed a definition for and the concept of disability, described the magnitude and dimensions of disability, and detailed a model for prevention. The authors did note that more nurses were needed to care for persons with IDD and that educational programs should include content on disabilities and care for this population. The second document was a follow-up to the first. The authors (Committee on Disability in America, Field, & Jette, 2007) provided a progress report that updated the 1991 document and recommended that more funding and attention be allocated to help healthcare consumers with disabilities, including IDD, to live their lives as optimally as possible given appropriate supports. Emphasis was placed on disability monitoring, research, and access to all needed health and additional support services. Again, the significance to nursing was the need for content and practice opportunities in educational programs so that graduates and experienced nurses entering into the IDD specialization would be prepared to care for this population.

Integrating the Science and Art of IDD Nursing

Like the profession of nursing, the nursing specialty of IDD is built on a core body of knowledge that reflects its components of science and art. Nursing in IDD requires judgment and skill based on biological, physical, behavioral, and social sciences. Nurses use critical thinking to apply the best available evidence and research data when responding to the needs of individuals with IDD, evaluating the quality and effectiveness of nursing practice, and seeking to optimize outcomes for individuals with IDD and their families/legal guardians.

The Science of IDD Nursing

The IDD nursing specialty is based on the nursing process, in which critical thinking is used to assess, diagnose, identify outcomes, plan, implement, and evaluate nursing care and outcomes of individuals with IDD. These steps serve as the foundation of clinical decision-making and support evidence-based practice. Nursing care in this specialty is defined by the standards of nursing practice and professional performance for nurses who specialize in IDD. The phenomena of concern to nurses who specialize in IDD center on individuals with IDD, their family/legal guardian, and the community (see Figure 3).

The Art of IDD Nursing

The art of nursing is based on caring and respect for human dignity. Nurses provide compassionate and competent care to individuals with IDD in independent practice and partnerships. Nurses collaborate with other colleagues and with individuals with IDD and their families/legal guardians to meet or help meet the needs of individuals with IDD.

FIGURE 3. Phenomena of Concern to Nurses Who Specialize in IDD

Individuals

- Adequate and appropriate primary health care and immunizations based on chronological age.
- Advocacy.
- Appropriate healthcare teaching at the individual's developmental level.
- Appropriate management of acute and chronic illnesses.
- Consistent and ongoing collaboration with the individual regarding management of health care, person-centered health care.
- Developing, implementing, and evaluating the Individualized Family Support Plan (IFSP), Individualized Education Plan (IEP), Individualized Health Plan (IHP), Individualized Plan for Employment (IPE), or Individualized Transition Plan (ITP) with an interprofessional team which includes the individual with IDD and their family members.
- Developmental interventions based on developmental and functional ability rather than chronological age.
- Holistic management of psychosocial concerns—caring for the whole person.
- Legal issues or concerns.
- Prevention of secondary disorders.
- Respect for cultural, religious, and socioeconomic differences.
- Unique anatomical, physiological, and psychological differences depending on diagnosis (e.g., genetic disorder, physical disability).

Family

- Advocacy.
- Continuous collaboration with family members regarding management of health care.
- Family-centered approach that is respectful of the family's culture, religion, and socioeconomic standing.

FIGURE 3. Continued

Community

- Care management across the individual's lifespan.
- Economic and political changes and their influence on financial status of the family (e.g., changes in Social Security services and benefits).
- Keeping up to date on advances in nursing and related professions involved in the care of individuals with IDD.
- Keeping up to date on political and policy changes and being able to translate these and communicate changes to individuals with IDD and their family.

The art of nursing in this specialty is dynamic and encompasses a holistic approach in providing care. To foster health and healing of the whole person, the nurse must be able to communicate effectively with individuals with IDD, who may have difficulty communicating through usual written or verbal channels. Thus, the nurse must have the skills to understand and interpret the signs and cues sent by individuals with IDD to communicate their needs and desires.

As in the profession of nursing, nursing in IDD aims to modify the impact of illness and disease on individuals with IDD, modify the relationship between individuals and their environment as needed to support the health of individuals with IDD, and promote healthy patterns of living. In addition to promoting and maintaining health and preventing or resolving disease and illness, IDD nursing aims to prevent further disability. When individuals with IDD have a disease and illness, nurses should be careful to distinguish signs and symptoms of the disease or illness from characteristics of the disability. This is especially important when an individual's disability manifests in ways that are similar to a disease or illness. Last, when planning and implementing care, nurses may have opportunities to develop innovative and creative approaches to assure positive outcomes for the individual with IDD and his or her family/legal guardian.

IDD Nursing's Societal and Ethical Dimensions

Intellectual and developmental disability nursing is responsive to the changing needs of society and the expanding knowledge base of its theoretical and scientific domains. One objective of nurses who specialize in IDD is to achieve positive outcomes that maximize quality of life across the entire lifespan. Registered nurses specializing in IDD facilitate the interprofessional and comprehensive care provided by healthcare professionals, paraprofessionals, and volunteers. In other instances, nurses consult with other colleagues to inform decision-making and planning to meet the healthcare needs of individuals with IDD. Registered nurses specializing in IDD participate in interprofessional teams in which the overlapping skills complement and enhance each member's individual efforts.

IDD nursing practice, like all nursing practice, is fundamentally independent practice. Registered nurses are accountable for nursing judgments made and actions taken in the course of their nursing practice. Therefore, the registered nurse specializing in IDD is responsible for assessing individual competence and is committed to the process of lifelong learning. Registered nurses specializing in IDD develop and maintain current knowledge and skills through formal and continuing education and seek available certification.

All registered nurses are bound by a professional code of ethics (ANA, 2001) and regulate themselves as individuals through a collegial process of peer review of practice. Peer evaluation fosters the refinement of knowledge, skills, and clinical decision-making at all levels and in IDD nursing practice. Self-regulation by the profession of nursing assures quality of performance, which is the heart of nursing's social contract (ANA, 2010b).

Registered nurses specializing in IDD nursing and members of various professions exchange knowledge and ideas about how to deliver high-quality health care, resulting in overlaps and constantly changing professional practice boundaries. This interprofessional team collaboration involves recognition of the expertise of others within and outside one's profession and referral to those providers when appropriate. Such collaboration also involves some shared functions and a common focus on one overall mission. By necessity, IDD nursing's scope of practice has flexible boundaries.

Registered nurses specializing in IDD regularly evaluate safety, effectiveness, and cost in the planning and delivery of nursing care to individuals with IDD. Nurses recognize that resources are limited and unequally distributed, and that the potential for improving access to care requires innovative approaches, such as treating individuals with IDD remotely. As members of a profession, registered nurses work toward equitable distribution and availability of healthcare services to individuals with IDD throughout the nation and the world.

Caring and IDD Nursing Practice

Consistent with Watson's Transpersonal Caring-Healing Framework (1999, 2008), the nurse defines the individual with IDD as a unique human being and stresses the importance of the connections between the nurse and the individual with IDD. There is an emphasis on the relationship between the nurse and the individual with IDD and the family. Nurses support the right of individuals with IDD to self-determination. That is, individuals with IDD have opportunities and experiences that enable them to have control in their lives and to advocate for themselves [Arc of the United States (ARC) & American Association on Intellectual and Developmental Disabilities (AAIDD), 2008b]. Individuals with IDD learn skills and have experiences that facilitate personal control over their health and lead to healthy choices. As self-advocates, individuals with IDD should be heard, respected, and supported to fully participate in their own health care. Nurses work to assure that individuals with IDD and their families have the knowledge and skills to engage in informed decision-making about health. Family members and substitute decision-makers may need assistance in understanding the importance of self-determination and the limits that self-determination can place on their own authority to make decisions with and for the individual with IDD.

The nurse provides care to individuals with IDD and their families/legal guardians in a manner that reflects sensitivity to culture and varied expressions of care among all cultures (Leininger, 1988), and supports the implementation of caring processes built on Watson's framework and described by Swanson (1993). Nurses (a) believe in individuals with IDD and their ability to move through events and transitions; (b) work to understand the meaning of health and health-related events from the perspective of individuals with IDD and their families/legal guardians; (c) are emotionally present for individuals with IDD and their families/legal guardians; (d) carry out health-related activities and tasks for individuals with IDD and their families/legal guardians when these persons cannot carry out these activities and tasks themselves; and

(e) support and facilitate transitions and unfamiliar events experienced by individuals with IDD and their families/legal guardians.

Nurses should be mindful that the experiences of individuals with IDD in society may be those of oppression and limitations on their ability to fully participate in their communities and be treated equally. Health services such as routine gynecological care, mammograms, and preventive and therapeutic dental services should be accessible to individuals with IDD. There should be a balance between undertreatment—the limitations of treatment based on IDD diagnosis—and overtreatment—the unwillingness to recognize when treatment is no longer beneficial. Nurses may have advocacy and educator roles in the decision-making process with the individual with IDD, if capable; the family, if appropriate; and others involved in the individual's care.

Advances in assistive and medical technology contribute to improved health, functioning ability, and quality of life in individuals with IDD. Assistive technology should benefit individuals with IDD by improving their independence, mobility, communication, and ability to control their environment (AAIDD & ARC, 2008). Medical technology should be directed toward improving quality of life and relieving pain, isolation, fear, and physical discomforts. Individuals with IDD should have the opportunity to accept or refuse services after they have been provided information and assisted to understand the risks and benefits of services. When information cannot be provided in a way that takes into account the communication and cognitive limitations of the individual with IDD to ensure informed consent, then the individual's advocate (i.e., guardian, health care power of attorney, or surrogate decision-maker; Midwest Bioethics Center & University of Missouri-Kansas City, 1996) should be involved to assure that the individual's demonstrations of acceptance or refusal are respected and followed (ARC & AAIDD, 2008a). Nurses should advocate for a careful evaluation of the benefits and risks of a proposed treatment for an individual with or at risk for IDD and not accept a categorical denial or plan to institute treatment based on another's estimation of the quality of life of the individual with or at risk for IDD.

Genetic and genomic advances promise both gains for and threats to individuals with IDD. Sometime in the future, the basis for IDD may be identified and eventually "treated" with gene therapy. If this technology evolves, there may be social pressure to submit to the treatment to ameliorate or eliminate the disability, and even less tolerance for the spectrum of human difference.

Some assume that if a prenatal disability is detected, the mother (or parents) will choose to terminate the pregnancy. Nurses respect the autonomous decisions of the mother, but also grant that the mother's decision may be influenced by society's response to individuals with IDD and tolerance for difference.

In addition to the significant ethical concerns and issues, nurses must be knowledgeable regarding psychological, social, economic, cultural, and legal issues. Nurses must grasp the interprofessional nature of health care in this field and be prepared to provide case management services to individuals with IDD.

Continued Commitment to the Profession of IDD Nursing

The nurse's practice in IDD is both independent and collaborative. The nurse's independent responsibility is assessment, the formulation of nursing diagnosis, the care of human responses to health and illness, and the evaluation of individual and family outcomes (ANA, 2010a). The guiding principles for nurses in providing services to individuals with IDD across the lifespan include:

- Collaborative, comprehensive, and coordinated care;

- Cultural competence;

- Developmental appropriateness;

- Family-/person-centered care;

- Inclusiveness; and

- Normalization.

Each of these terms is defined in the glossary. Nurses in IDD further provide services that incorporate system assessment, policy development and implementation, and quality assurance, and support the medical home concept.

Nurses are committed to this specialty because their passion is the care of individuals with IDD. There are many challenges and rewards in this field. Advances in science, especially in genetics and diagnostic technology, provide new insights and understanding of different conditions, their etiology, their trajectory, possible secondary conditions, and strategies for the management of the individual's health care so that quality of life can become and remain optimal. Learning about and caring for individuals with IDD often enlighten and add meaning to one's nursing care.

Nurses who specialize in this field learn that they are more alike than different. Nurses learn to appreciate an individual's strengths and assist the individual to maximize these strengths and function within existing limits. Challenges may include (a) a multitude of health problems that require many treatments or medications; (b) uncertainty regarding the future, because healthcare professionals do not know all there is to know about these conditions across the lifespan, and especially in middle and late adulthood; and (c) frustration with a society that views individuals with IDD as different. This nursing specialty is critical to health care, as there always will be individuals with IDD who need nursing professionals who care about and for their healthcare needs.

Nurses in this field must engage in continuous learning to improve and strengthen their practice in whatever practice setting. Nurses at any level of practice must also be active in nursing and specialty organizations at local, regional, national, or international levels. Nursing leadership is important in these organizations at all levels, as well as in the communities. The code of ethics (ANA, 2001) serves as the ethical framework in nursing regardless of practice setting or role, and provides guidance for the future.

Professional Trends and Issues in IDD Nursing

Currently, nurses in IDD are involved through their practice and advocacy in a number of issues: predominant cultural concerns, early assessment and identification, inclusion in the school and community, adult health care and chronic disease conditions, transition from pediatric to adult healthcare services, self-advocacy and self-determination, employment, community living, limited healthcare resources, and genetics. As nurses care for individuals with IDD and their families/legal guardians from diverse backgrounds, culturally competent methods of communication, care, and intervention must be developed and evaluated.

Nurses play a key role in the healthcare management of the individual with IDD throughout the individual's life. Especially important is the transition from pediatric to adult healthcare services, during which nurses must help ensure that individuals with IDD living in a variety of residential settings, including the biological home, receive regular, quality health care, and that adolescents and adults with IDD learn to advocate for themselves. New discoveries in genetics have created vast opportunities for nurses to improve identification of the need for services; coordination of services; referral for further evaluation; education; identification, prevention, and management of primary and secondary disease conditions; and evaluation and follow-up of such conditions.

There is also a nursing shortage in this specialty. Efforts are being made in public and private agencies to increase salaries. Nursing organizations develop continuing education and distance learning projects, as well as a core curriculum to assist nurses in learning more about IDD and the needed nursing care (Nehring, 2010). Nurses, across time, have contributed to the field by writing books, articles, and pamphlets; directing films; and producing Internet and distance learning products to illustrate best practices and evidence-based care for nurses. Integration of IDD content into entry-level nursing curricula is needed to ensure that registered nurses have the basic knowledge and skills to provide safe and competent care to this population.

Summary of the Scope of IDD Nursing Practice

The dynamic nature of the healthcare practice environment and the growing body of nursing research provide both the impetus and the opportunity for nursing in IDD to ensure competent nursing practice in all settings for all individuals with IDD and to promote ongoing professional development that enhances the quality of nursing practice. *Intellectual and Developmental Disabilities Nursing: Scope and Standards of Practice, Second Edition*, assists that process by delineating the professional scope and standards of practice and responsibilities of all professional registered nurses engaged in IDD nursing practice, regardless of setting. As such, it can serve as a basis for:

- Quality improvement systems

- Regulatory systems

- Healthcare reimbursement and financing methodologies

- Development and evaluation of nursing service delivery systems and organizational structures

- Certification activities

- Position descriptions and performance appraisals

- Agency policies, procedures, and protocols

- Educational offerings

- Establishing the legal standard of care

Standards of Professional Nursing Practice for Intellectual and Developmental Disabilities (IDD) Nurses

Significance of Standards for IDD Nurses

The Standards of Professional Nursing Practice are authoritative statements of the duties that all registered nurses, regardless of role, population, or specialty, are expected to perform competently. The standards published herein may be utilized as evidence of the standard of care, with the understanding that application of the standards is context dependent. The standards are subject to change with the dynamics of the nursing profession, as new patterns of professional practice are developed and accepted by the nursing profession and the public. In addition, specific conditions and clinical circumstances may also affect the application of the standards at a given time (e.g., during a natural disaster). The standards are subject to formal, periodic review and revision.

The competencies that accompany each standard may be evidence of compliance with the corresponding standard. The list of competencies is not exhaustive. Whether a particular standard or competency applies depends upon the circumstances.

These standards apply to both the registered nurse and APRN in IDD. They apply to the nursing care of persons with IDD of all ages, cultures, socioeconomic backgrounds, and medical diagnoses. Furthermore, these standards apply to any health care, education, residential, or community setting where healthcare consumers with IDD might be. The competencies have been developed by the authors to represent quality practice and performance in the nursing care of healthcare consumers with IDD.

Standards of Practice for IDD Nurses

Standard 1. Assessment

The registered nurse who specializes in IDD collects comprehensive data pertinent to the healthcare consumer's health and/or the situation.

COMPETENCIES
The registered nurse:

- Collects comprehensive data including but not limited to physical, functional, psychosocial, emotional, cognitive, sexual, cultural, age-related, environmental, spiritual/transpersonal, and economic assessments in a systematic and ongoing process while honoring the uniqueness of the person. This may involve observation, interviewing, and the use of screening and assessment tools. Diagnostic tests may be used as part of the assessment process if the nurse has specific training in that area (e.g., developmental diagnostic testing).

- Uses analytical models and problem-solving tools that are appropriate for healthcare consumers with IDD.

- Elicits the values, preferences, expressed needs, and knowledge of the healthcare situation of the consumer with IDD and family/legal guardians.

- Involves the healthcare consumer with IDD, family/legal guardians, other healthcare and interdisciplinary professionals and paraprofessionals, and the work and home environment, as appropriate, in holistic data collection.

- Identifies barriers (e.g., cognitive, physical, psychosocial, literacy, financial, cultural) to effective communication and makes appropriate adaptations.

- Recognizes the impact of personal attitudes, values, and beliefs.

- Assesses family dynamics and impact on health and wellness of the consumer with IDD.

- Prioritizes data collection based on the immediate condition or the anticipated needs of the healthcare consumer with IDD or situation.

- Uses appropriate evidence-based assessment techniques, instruments, and tools in collecting pertinent data, including, but not limited to, genetic studies, special serum screening (e.g., cystic fibrosis, Tay-Sachs, sickle-cell disease), nutritional needs and metabolic functioning, and any other condition-specific data measures.

- Synthesizes all data, information, and knowledge from the consumer with IDD, family members/legal guardians, the interdisciplinary team, and the individual's environment that is relevant to the situation to identify patterns and variances. This may involve data and information from the school, work site, and/or residential setting.

- Applies ethical, legal, and privacy guidelines and policies to the collection, maintenance, use, and dissemination of data and information.

- Recognizes that healthcare consumers with IDD have authority over their own health by honoring their care preferences. As legally appropriate, a guardian may be involved in identifying and expressing those preferences.

- Documents relevant data in a retrievable format.

ADDITIONAL COMPETENCIES FOR THE
APRN WHO SPECIALIZES IN IDD

The advanced practice registered nurse:

- Initiates and interprets diagnostic tests and procedures relevant to the current status of the healthcare consumer with IDD.

- Assesses the effect of interactions among individuals, family/legal guardians, community, and social systems on health and illness.

Standard 2. Diagnosis

The registered nurse who specializes in IDD analyzes the assessment data to determine the diagnoses or issues.

COMPETENCIES

The registered nurse:

- Derives the diagnoses or issues from assessment data.

- Validates the diagnoses or issues in partnership with the healthcare consumer with IDD, family/legal guardians, and members of the interdisciplinary team when possible and appropriate.

- Identifies actual or potential risks to the health and safety of the consumer with IDD or barriers to health, which may include but are not limited to interpersonal, systematic, or environmental circumstances.

- Uses standardized classification systems and clinical decision support tools, when available, in identifying diagnoses.

- Documents diagnoses or issues in a manner that facilitates the determination of the expected outcomes and plan.

ADDITIONAL COMPETENCIES FOR THE
APRN WHO SPECIALIZES IN IDD

The advanced practice registered nurse:

- Systematically compares and contrasts the history and clinical findings with normal and abnormal variations and developmental events in formulating differential diagnoses, including specific values, ranges, and outcomes for a specific diagnosis (e.g., Down syndrome).

- Synthesizes complex data and information (including developmental and assessment) obtained during interview, examination, and diagnostic processes when identifying diagnoses.

■ Serves as a consultant to the registered nurse and other staff in developing and maintaining competence in the diagnostic process.

■ Analyzes accessibility and availability of services, barriers to adequate health care, specific populations at high risk, health promotion needs for specific populations, and environmental hazards that may affect health.

Standard 3. Outcomes Identification

The registered nurse who specializes in IDD identifies expected outcomes for a plan individualized to the healthcare consumer with IDD or the situation.

COMPETENCIES

The registered nurse:

- Partners with the healthcare consumer with IDD, family/legal guardians, members of the interprofessional team, and others in formulating expected outcomes when possible and appropriate.

- Derives culturally appropriate expected outcomes from the diagnoses.

- Considers associated risks, benefits, costs, current scientific evidence, expected trajectory of the condition, and clinical expertise when formulating expected outcomes.

- Defines expected outcomes in terms of the values of the healthcare consumer with IDD; the values of family members/legal guardians when appropriate; ethical and legal considerations; environment, culture, or situation with such consideration as associated risks; benefits and costs; and current scientific, ethical, and/or legal evidence.

- Develops expected outcomes that facilitate continuity of care and person-centered care as appropriate.

- Modifies expected outcomes according to changes in the status (i.e., health, social, living, economic, and/or legal) of the healthcare consumer with IDD or evaluation of the situation.

- Documents expected outcomes as measurable goals that include an estimated time to attain expected outcomes.

ADDITIONAL COMPETENCIES FOR THE
APRN WHO SPECIALIZES IN IDD

The advanced practice registered nurse:

- Identifies expected outcomes that incorporate scientific evidence and are achievable through implementation of evidence-based practices.

- Identifies expected outcomes that incorporate cost and clinical effectiveness, legal and ethical boundaries, satisfaction and understanding, and consistency and continuity among the individual with IDD, family/legal guardians, healthcare providers, and members of the interprofessional team.

- Supports the use of clinical guidelines linked to positive patient outcomes.

- Differentiates outcomes that require care process interventions from those that require system-level interventions.

Standard 4. Planning

The registered nurse who specializes in IDD develops a plan that prescribes strategies and alternatives to attain expected outcomes.

COMPETENCIES

The registered nurse:

- Develops an individualized plan that is person-centered when appropriate, in partnership with the person, family/legal guardians, and others considering the person's characteristics or situation, including but not limited to values, beliefs, spiritual and health practices, preferences, choices, chronological age and developmental level, coping style, culture, available technology, and the least restrictive environment.

- Establishes the plan priorities in collaboration with the healthcare consumer with IDD, family/legal guardians, others, and the interprofessional team as appropriate.

- Includes strategies in the plan that address each of the identified diagnoses or issues. These strategies may include but are not limited to strategies for:

  - Promotion and restoration of health;

  - Prevention of illness, injury, and disease;

  - Alleviation of suffering; and

  - Supportive care for those who are dying.

- Includes strategies for health and wholeness across the lifespan.

- Provides for continuity in the plan.

- Incorporates an implementation pathway or timeline in the plan.

- Considers the economic impact of the plan on the healthcare consumer with IDD, family/legal guardians, caregivers, or other affected parties.

- Integrates current scientific evidence, trends, and research affecting comprehensive care of healthcare consumers of all ages with IDD into the planning process.

- Uses the plan to provide direction to family members/legal guardians and other members of the healthcare and interprofessional team.

- Investigates practice settings and safe space and time for the nurse and the healthcare consumer with IDD to explore suggested, potential, and alternative options.

- Defines the plan to reflect current statutes, rules and regulations, and standards.

- Modifies the plan according to the ongoing assessment of the healthcare consumer's response and other outcome indicators.

- Documents the plan in a manner that uses standardized, person-first language and recognized terminology.

ADDITIONAL COMPETENCIES FOR THE APRN WHO SPECIALIZES IN IDD

The advanced practice registered nurse:

- Identifies assessment strategies, screening and diagnostic strategies, and therapeutic interventions that reflect current evidence, including data, research, literature, and expert clinical knowledge.

- Selects or designs strategies to meet the multifaceted and complex needs of healthcare consumers with IDD.

- Includes in the plan a synthesis of the values and beliefs of the healthcare consumer with IDD regarding nursing, medical, social, and educational therapies.

- Leads the design and development of interprofessional processes to address the identified diagnosis, situation, or issue.

- Actively participates in the development and continuous improvement of organizational systems that support the planning process.

- Supports the integration of clinical, human, and financial resources to enhance and complete the decision-making and evaluation processes.

- Serves as a consultant to the registered nurse in plan development, priority setting, cost-benefit analysis, and identification of resources, as needed.

- In collaboration with the registered nurse and other members of the interprofessional team, and in partnership with the community, derives community-focused plans that are based on identified problems, conditions, or needs and that build on the strengths of the community.

- Develops plans that ensure continuity of care and minimize or eliminate gaps and duplication of services.

Standard 5. Implementation

The registered nurse who specializes in IDD implements the identified plan.

COMPETENCIES
The registered nurse:

- Partners with the healthcare consumer with IDD, his or her family/legal guardians, significant others, and caregivers as appropriate to implement the plan in a safe, realistic, and timely manner.

- Demonstrates caring behaviors toward healthcare consumers with IDD, significant others, and groups of people receiving care.

- Utilizes technology to measure, record, and retrieve healthcare consumer data, implement the nursing process, and enhance nursing practice.

- Utilizes evidence-based interventions and treatments specific to the diagnosis or problem.

- Provides holistic care that addresses the needs of diverse populations across the lifespan.

- Advocates for health care that is sensitive to the needs of healthcare consumers with IDD, with particular emphasis on the needs of diverse populations.

- Applies appropriate knowledge of major health problems and cultural diversity in implementing the plan of care.

- Applies available healthcare technologies to maximize access and optimize outcomes for healthcare consumers with IDD.

- Utilizes community resources and systems to implement the plan.

- Collaborates with nursing colleagues and other healthcare providers from diverse backgrounds to implement and integrate the plan.

- Accommodates different styles of communication used by healthcare consumers with IDD, families/legal guardians, members of the interdisciplinary team, and other healthcare providers.

- Integrates traditional and complementary healthcare practices as appropriate.

- Implements the plan in a timely manner in accordance with patient safety goals.

- Promotes the capacity of the healthcare consumer with IDD to achieve the optimal level of participation and problem-solving.

- Documents implementation of and any modifications, including changes or omissions, to the identified plan.

ADDITIONAL COMPETENCIES FOR THE
APRN WHO SPECIALIZES IN IDD

The advanced practice registered nurse:

- Facilitates utilization of systems, organizations, and community resources to implement the plan.

- Supports collaboration with nursing colleagues and other members of the interprofessional team to implement the plan.

- Incorporates new knowledge and strategies to initiate change in nursing care practices if desired outcomes are not achieved.

- Assumes responsibility for safe and efficient implementation of the plan.

- Uses advanced communication skills to promote relationships between nurses and healthcare consumers with IDD, to provide a context for open communication about the healthcare consumer's experiences, and to improve healthcare consumer outcomes.

- Actively participates in the development and continuous improvement of systems that support implementation of the plan.

- Implements the plan using principles and concepts of project or systems management.

- Fosters organizational systems that support implementation of the plan.

Standard 5A. Coordination of Care

The registered nurse who specializes in IDD coordinates care delivery.

COMPETENCIES

The registered nurse:

- Organizes the components of the healthcare plan.

- Manages the care for a healthcare consumer with IDD to maximize independence and quality of life.

- Assists the healthcare consumer with IDD and the family/legal guardians, as appropriate, to identify options for alternative care.

- Communicates with the healthcare consumer with IDD, family/legal guardians, and system during transitions in care.

- Advocates for the delivery of dignified and humane care by the interprofessional team.

- Documents the coordination of care.

- Makes referrals to other disciplines as needed.

- Supervises and/or provides direction to ancillary and unlicensed personnel who provide health care to healthcare consumers with IDD and their families/legal guardians.

- Keeps the healthcare consumer with IDD and family/legal guardians (and direct care support professionals, when present) informed about the health status of the consumer.

- Keeps the healthcare consumer and the family/legal guardians informed about healthcare resources that are available.

- Employs strategies to promote health in home and community settings that are safe and utilize the least restrictive alternatives.

ADDITIONAL COMPETENCIES FOR THE
APRN WHO SPECIALIZES IN IDD

The advanced practice registered nurse:

- Provides leadership in the coordination of interprofessional health care for integrated delivery of healthcare services for the healthcare consumer with IDD.

- Synthesizes data and information to prescribe necessary system and community support measures, including modifications of surroundings.

- Coordinates system and community resources that enhance delivery of care across continuums.

Standard 5B. Health Teaching and Health Promotion

The registered nurse who specializes in IDD employs strategies to promote health and a safe environment.

COMPETENCIES

The registered nurse:

- Provides health teaching that addresses such topics as healthy lifestyles, risk-reducing behaviors, developmental needs, activities of daily living, self-care concepts, and preventive self-care.

- Uses health promotion and health teaching methods that are appropriate to the situation and that recognize the values, beliefs, health practices, developmental level, learning needs, readiness and ability to learn, language preference, spirituality, culture, and socioeconomic status of the healthcare consumer with IDD.

- Seeks opportunities for feedback and evaluation of the effectiveness of the strategies used.

- Uses information technologies to communicate health promotion and disease prevention information to healthcare consumers with IDD and their families/legal guardians in a variety of settings.

- Provides healthcare consumers with IDD and their families/legal guardians with information about intended effects and potential adverse effects of proposed therapies.

ADDITIONAL COMPETENCIES FOR THE
APRN WHO SPECIALIZES IN IDD

The advanced practice registered nurse:

- Synthesizes empirical evidence on risk behaviors, learning theories, behavioral change theories, motivational theories, epidemiology, and other related theories and frameworks when designing health education information and programs.

■ Conducts personalized health teaching and counseling considering comparative effectiveness research recommendations.

■ Designs health information and healthcare consumer education appropriate to the developmental level, learning needs, readiness to learn, and cultural values and beliefs of the healthcare consumer with IDD.

■ Evaluates health information resources, such as the Internet, within the area of practice for accuracy, readability, and comprehensibility to help healthcare consumers with IDD, family/legal guardians, and other members of the interprofessional team access quality health information.

■ Engages consumer alliances and advocacy groups, as appropriate, in health teaching and health promotion activities.

■ Provides anticipatory guidance to individuals with IDD, families/legal guardians, groups, and communities to promote health and prevent or reduce the risk of health problems.

Standard 5C. Consultation

The advanced practice registered nurse who specializes in IDD provides consultation to influence the identified plan, enhance the abilities of others, and effect change.

COMPETENCIES FOR THE APRN WHO SPECIALIZES IN IDD
The advanced practice registered nurse:

- Synthesizes clinical data, theoretical frameworks, and evidence when providing consultation.

- Facilitates the effectiveness of a consultation by involving the healthcare consumer with IDD, family/legal guardians, and other stakeholders in decision-making and negotiating role responsibilities.

- Communicates consultation recommendations that influence the plan of care, facilitate understanding by involving stakeholders, enhance the work of others, and effect change.

- Influences health and social policies that affect healthcare consumers with IDD.

Standard 5D. Prescriptive Authority and Treatment

The advanced practice registered nurse who specializes in IDD uses prescriptive authority, procedures, referrals, treatments, and therapies in accordance with state and federal laws and regulations.

COMPETENCIES FOR THE APRN WHO SPECIALIZES IN IDD
The advanced practice registered nurse:

- Prescribes evidence-based treatments, therapies, and procedures considering the comprehensive healthcare needs of the healthcare consumer with IDD.

- Prescribes pharmacologic agents according to a current knowledge of pharmacology and physiology.

- Prescribes specific pharmacologic agents or treatments based on clinical indicators, the needs and status of the healthcare consumer with IDD, and the results of diagnostic and laboratory tests.

- Evaluates therapeutic and potential adverse effects of pharmacologic and nonpharmacologic treatments.

- Provides healthcare consumers with IDD with information about intended effects and potential adverse effects of proposed prescriptive therapies.

- Provides information about costs and alternative treatments and procedures, as appropriate.

- Evaluates and incorporates complementary and alternative therapy into education and practice.

Standard 6: Evaluation

The registered nurse who specializes in IDD evaluates progress toward attainment of outcomes.

COMPETENCIES

The registered nurse:

- Conducts a systematic, ongoing, and criterion-based evaluation of outcomes in relation to the structures and processes prescribed by the plan of care and the indicated timeline.

- Collaborates with the healthcare consumer with IDD, his or her family/legal guardians, members of the interprofessional team, and others involved in the care or situation in the evaluation process.

- Evaluates, in partnership with the healthcare consumer with IDD and members of the interprofessional team, the effectiveness of the planned strategies in relation to the healthcare consumer's responses and attainment of the expected outcomes.

- Uses ongoing assessment data to revise the diagnoses, outcomes, the plan, and the implementation as needed.

- Disseminates the results of the evaluation to the healthcare consumer with IDD and others involved in the care or situation, as appropriate, in accordance with federal and state regulations.

- Participates in assessing and assuring the responsible and appropriate use of interventions in order to minimize unwarranted or unwanted treatment and healthcare consumer suffering.

- Documents the results of the evaluation.

ADDITIONAL COMPETENCIES FOR THE
APRN WHO SPECIALIZES IN IDD

The advanced practice registered nurse:

- Evaluates the accuracy of the diagnosis and the effectiveness of the interventions and other variables in relation to the attainment of expected outcomes.

- Synthesizes the results of the evaluation to determine the effect of the plan on healthcare consumers with IDD, families/legal guardians, groups, communities, and institutions.

- Adapts the plan of care for the trajectory of treatment according to evaluation of response.

- Uses the results of the evaluation to make or recommend process or structural changes, including policy, procedure, or protocol revision, as appropriate.

Standards of Professional Performance for IDD Nurses

Standard 7. Ethics

The registered nurse who specializes in IDD practices ethically.

COMPETENCIES

The registered nurse:

- Uses *Code of Ethics for Nurses with Interpretive Statements* (ANA, 2001) to guide practice.

- Delivers care in a manner that preserves and protects the autonomy, dignity, rights, values, and beliefs of the healthcare consumer with IDD.

- Recognizes the centrality of the healthcare consumer with IDD and family/legal guardians as core members of any healthcare team.

- Upholds confidentiality of the healthcare consumer with IDD within legal and regulatory parameters.

- Serves as advocate for the healthcare consumer with IDD and family/ legal guardians by supporting the development of their advocacy and self-advocacy skills.

- Maintains a therapeutic and professional relationship with the healthcare consumer with IDD within appropriate professional role boundaries.

- Contributes to resolving ethical issues involving the healthcare consumer with IDD, colleagues, community groups, systems, and other stakeholders as evidenced by activities such as participating on ethics committees.

- Takes appropriate action regarding instances of illegal, unethical, or inappropriate behavior that can endanger or jeopardize the best interests of the healthcare consumer with IDD or situation.

- Speaks up to question healthcare practice when necessary for safety and quality improvement.

- Advocates for equitable healthcare consumer care.

- Participates on interprofessional teams that address ethical risks, benefits, and outcomes.

- Informs administrators or others of the risks, benefits, and outcomes of programs and decisions that affect healthcare delivery.

- Respects the right of the healthcare consumer with IDD to self-determination and includes the healthcare consumer in decisions unless the healthcare consumer's incapacity to participate in a specific decision is demonstrated. Family or a legally designated guardian is included in decision-making or makes the decision as a surrogate decision-maker if legally required.

- Identifies a surrogate for healthcare decisions in lieu of a formal guardianship process, when appropriate and in accordance with local and/or state statutes.

- Advocates for the healthcare consumer with IDD in self-determination decisions when in conflict with the surrogate decision-maker.

- Facilitates the self-determination decisions of the healthcare consumer with IDD in all healthcare settings.

- Acts as an advocate for the healthcare consumer with IDD and family/legal guardian and initiates referral to a qualified advocate for healthcare consumers with IDD when appropriate.

- Works to prevent abuse or exploitation of the healthcare consumer with IDD and promptly responds to suspicion or evidence by reporting to appropriate authorities.

- Assists in assuring that the living arrangement for the healthcare consumer with IDD is the most appropriate and least restrictive environment.

- Contributes to the educational program recommendations and advocates for the least restrictive environment to maximize the potential of the healthcare consumer with IDD.

- Contributes to the life plan and advocates for the most appropriate employment situation for the healthcare consumer with IDD. The nurse assists in identifying reasonable accommodations to maximize the healthcare consumer's performance and satisfaction with chosen employment.

- Assists in the referral process for local, state, regional, and federal assistance programs.

- Supports the expression of sexuality of the healthcare consumer with IDD in a manner that is consistent with the healthcare consumer's native culture, religious upbringing, family values, and level of maturity and provides counseling as appropriate.

- Contributes to an environment that protects the healthcare consumer with IDD from sexual exploitation at home, school, work, and community.

- Serves as an advocate to ensure that the healthcare consumer with IDD receives coordinated, continuous, and accessible health care that is provided by a professional who is competent in managing health concerns of healthcare consumers with IDD.

- Educates colleagues outside of the IDD specialty who provide health care to healthcare consumers with IDD.

- Provides support and resources for end-of-life care, grief, and bereavement when healthcare consumers with IDD experience loss.

- Provides or arranges for effective and appropriate palliative care for healthcare consumers with IDD who undergo tests or treatments for illnesses, have chronic conditions, and/or are at the end of life.

- Advocates for life-sustaining treatment or refusal/withdrawal of life-sustaining treatment as the healthcare consumer with IDD and family or legal guardian decide.

- Demonstrates a commitment to practicing self-care, managing stress, and connecting with self and others.

ADDITIONAL COMPETENCIES FOR THE APRN WHO SPECIALIZES IN IDD

The advanced practice registered nurse:

- Informs the healthcare consumer with IDD and family/legal guardians of the risks, benefits, and outcomes of healthcare regimens to allow informed decision-making, including informed consent and informed refusal.

Standard 8. Education

The registered nurse who specializes in IDD attains knowledge and competence that reflect current nursing practice.

COMPETENCIES

The registered nurse:

- Participates in ongoing educational activities related to appropriate knowledge bases and professional issues.

- Demonstrates a commitment to lifelong learning through self-reflection and inquiry to address learning needs and personal growth needs.

- Seeks experiences that reflect current practice to maintain knowledge, skills, abilities, and judgment in clinical practice or role performance.

- Acquires knowledge and skills appropriate to the role, population, specialty, setting, role, or situation.

- Seeks formal and independent learning experiences to develop and maintain clinical and professional skills and knowledge.

- Identifies learning needs based on nursing knowledge, the various roles the nurse may assume, and the changing needs of the population.

- Participates in formal or informal consultations to address issues in nursing practice as an application of education and a knowledge base.

- Shares educational findings, experiences, and ideas with peers.

- Contributes to a work environment conducive to the education of healthcare professionals.

- Maintains professional records that provide evidence of competence and lifelong learning.

- Uses current healthcare research findings and other evidence related to the care of healthcare consumers with IDD to expand knowledge, skills, abilities, and judgment; to enhance role performance; and to increase knowledge of professional issues related to IDD nursing.

Standard 9. Evidence-Based Practice and Research

The registered nurse who specializes in IDD integrates evidence and research findings into practice.

COMPETENCIES

The registered nurse:

- Utilizes current evidence-based nursing knowledge, including research findings, to guide practice.

- Incorporates evidence when initiating changes in nursing practice.

- Participates, as appropriate to education level and position, in the formulation of evidence-based practice through research.

- Shares personal or third-party research findings with colleagues and peers.

- Participates, as appropriate to education level and position, in research activities to improve the health and health care of healthcare consumers with IDD.

- Engages healthcare consumers with IDD and their families/legal guardians in research activities consistent with their informed consent and informed refusal.

ADDITIONAL COMPETENCIES FOR THE APRN WHO SPECIALIZES IN IDD

The advanced practice registered nurse:

- Contributes to nursing knowledge by conducting or synthesizing research and other evidence that discovers, examines, and evaluates current practice, knowledge, theories, criteria, and creative approaches to improve healthcare outcomes of healthcare consumers with IDD.

- Promotes a climate of research and clinical inquiry.

- Disseminates research findings through activities such as presentations, publications, consultation, and journal clubs.

Standard 10. Quality of Practice

The registered nurse who specializes in IDD contributes to quality nursing practice.

COMPETENCIES

The registered nurse:

- Demonstrates quality nursing care by documenting the application of the nursing process in a responsible, accountable, and ethical manner.

- Uses creativity and innovation to enhance nursing care of healthcare consumers with IDD and their families/legal guardians.

- Participates in quality improvement. Activities may include:

  - Identifying aspects of practice important for quality monitoring;

  - Using indicators to monitor quality, safety, and effectiveness of nursing practice;

  - Collecting data to monitor quality and effectiveness of nursing practice;

  - Analyzing quality data to identify opportunities for improving nursing practice;

  - Formulating recommendations to improve nursing practice or outcomes;

  - Implementing activities to enhance the quality of nursing practice;

  - Developing, implementing, and/or evaluating policies, procedures, and guidelines to improve the quality of practice;

  - Participating on and/or leading interprofessional teams to evaluate clinical care or health services;

  - Participating in and/or leading efforts to minimize costs and unnecessary duplication;

- Identifying problems that occur in day-to-day work routines in order to correct process inefficiencies*;

- Analyzing factors related to quality, safety, and effectiveness;

- Analyzing organizational systems for barriers to quality healthcare outcomes of healthcare consumers with IDD; and

- Implementing processes to remove or weaken barriers within organizational systems.

- Provides leadership in the implementation of quality improvements for healthcare consumers with IDD and their families/legal guardians.

- Designs innovations to effect change in practice and improve health outcomes of healthcare consumers with IDD.

- Participates in the evaluation of the practice environment and quality of nursing care provided to healthcare consumers with IDD and their families/legal guardians.

- Evaluates nursing care delegated to other professionals, direct care support professionals, unlicensed assistive personnel, or the family/legal guardians and monitors health outcomes of the healthcare consumer with IDD.

- Identifies opportunities for the generation and use of research and evidence in IDD nursing.

- Participates in professional organizations that strive to improve the quality of nursing and health care provided to healthcare consumers with IDD and their families/legal guardians.

ADDITIONAL COMPETENCIES FOR THE APRN WHO SPECIALIZES IN IDD

The advanced practice registered nurse:

- Provides leadership in the design and implementation of quality improvements.

---

* Board of Higher Education/Massachusetts Organization of Nurse Executives (BHE/MONE), 2006.

- Evaluates the practice environment and quality of nursing care rendered in relation to existing evidence.

- Identifies opportunities for the generation and use of research and evidence.

- Obtains and maintains professional certification, as needed.

- Uses the results of quality improvement to initiate changes in nursing practice and the healthcare delivery system.

Standard 11. Communication

The registered nurse who specializes in IDD communicates effectively in a variety of formats in all areas of practice.

COMPETENCIES

The registered nurse:

- Assesses communication format preferences of healthcare consumers, families/legal guardians, and colleagues.*

- Assesses her or his own communication skills in encounters with healthcare consumers, families/legal guardians, and colleagues.*

- Seeks continuous improvement of her or his own communication and conflict resolution skills.*

- Conveys information to healthcare consumers, families/legal guardians, the interprofessional team, and others in communication formats that promote accuracy.

- Questions the rationale supporting care processes and decisions when they do not appear to be in the best interest of the healthcare consumer.*

- Discloses observations or concerns related to hazards and errors in care or the practice environment to the appropriate level.

- Maintains communication with other providers to minimize risks associated with transfers and transition in care delivery.

- Contributes her or his own professional perspective in discussions with the interprofessional team.

- Uses current knowledge of the adaptive and communication skills of the healthcare consumer with IDD to communicate effectively with the healthcare consumer.

- Facilitates communication between the healthcare consumer with IDD, family/legal guardians, and members of the interprofessional team, building on the adaptive and communication strengths of the healthcare consumer with IDD.

*BHE/MONE, 2006.

Standard 12. Leadership

The registered nurse who specializes in IDD demonstrates leadership in the professional practice setting and the profession.

COMPETENCIES

The registered nurse:

- Oversees the nursing care given by others while retaining accountability for the quality of care given to the healthcare consumer with IDD.

- Abides by the vision, the associated goals, and the plan to implement and measure progress of a healthcare consumer with IDD or progress within the context of the healthcare organization.

- Demonstrates a commitment to continuous, lifelong learning and education for self and others.

- Mentors colleagues for the advancement of nursing practice, the profession, and quality health care.

- Treats colleagues with respect, trust, and dignity.*

- Develops communication and conflict resolution skills.

- Participates in professional organizations.

- Communicates effectively with the healthcare consumer with IDD and colleagues.

- Seeks ways to advance nursing autonomy and accountability.*

- Participates in efforts to influence healthcare policy involving healthcare consumers with IDD and the profession.

- Influences decision-making bodies to improve the professional practice environment and healthcare outcomes of healthcare consumers with IDD and their families/legal guardians.

*BHE/MONE, 2006.

- Provides direction to enhance the effectiveness of the interprofessional team.

- Interprets the role of nursing for healthcare consumers with IDD, families/legal guardians, and others.

- Promotes communication of information and advancement of the profession as it relates to nursing and the field of IDD through writing, publishing, and presentation for professional or lay audiences.

- Designs innovations to effect change in IDD nursing practice and outcomes.

ADDITIONAL COMPETENCIES FOR THE APRN WHO SPECIALIZES IN IDD

The advanced practice registered nurse:

- Influences decision-making bodies to improve the professional practice environment and healthcare outcomes for healthcare consumers with IDD.

- Provides direction to enhance the effectiveness of the interprofessional team.

- Promotes advanced practice nursing and role development by interpreting its role for healthcare consumers with IDD, families/legal guardians, and others.

- Models expert practice to interprofessional team members and healthcare consumers with IDD.

- Mentors colleagues in the acquisition of clinical knowledge, skills, abilities, and judgment.

Standard 13. Collaboration

The registered nurse who specializes in IDD collaborates with the healthcare consumer with IDD, family/legal guardians, and others in the conduct of nursing practice.

COMPETENCIES
The registered nurse:

- Partners with others to effect change and produce positive outcomes through the sharing of knowledge of the healthcare consumer and/or situation.

- Communicates with the healthcare consumer with IDD, family/legal guardians, members of the interprofessional team, healthcare providers, and community providers regarding healthcare consumer care and the nurse's role in the provision of care.

- Promotes conflict management and engagement.

- Participates in building consensus or resolving conflict in the context of patient care.

- Applies group process and negotiation techniques with the healthcare consumer with IDD and colleagues.

- Adheres to standards and applicable codes of conduct that govern behavior among peers and colleagues to create a work environment that promotes cooperation, respect, and trust.

- Cooperates in creating a documented plan focused on outcomes and decisions related to care and delivery of services that indicates communication with healthcare consumers with IDD, families/legal guardians, and others.

- Engages in teamwork and team-building processes.

- Partners with other disciplines to enhance the outcomes of care of healthcare consumers with IDD through interprofessional activities, such as education, consultation, management, technological development, or research opportunities.

■ Documents plans, communications, rationales for plan changes, and collaborative discussions.

■ Partners with the healthcare consumer with IDD and family/legal guardians or significant others, and supports the efforts of healthcare consumers and family/legal guardians to make appropriate decisions about utilization of resources.

ADDITIONAL COMPETENCIES FOR THE APRN WHO SPECIALIZES IN IDD

The advanced practice registered nurse:

■ Partners with other disciplines to enhance the care of healthcare consumers with IDD through interprofessional activities, such as education, consultation, management, technological development, or research opportunities.

■ Invites the contribution of the healthcare consumer with IDD, family/legal guardians, and team members in order to achieve optimal outcomes.

■ Leads in establishing, improving, and sustaining collaborative relationships to achieve safe, quality health care.

■ Documents communications regarding the plan of care, rationales for changes to the plan, and collaborative discussions to improve the care of healthcare consumers with IDD.

■ Partners with other interprofessional administrative team members in policy-making and in overall agency and community planning, implementation, and evaluation of services to and programs for healthcare consumers with IDD.

Standard 14. Professional Practice Evaluation

The registered nurse who specializes in IDD evaluates her or his own nursing practice in relation to professional practice standards and guidelines, relevant statutes, rules, and regulations.

COMPETENCIES

The registered nurse:

- Provides age-appropriate and developmentally appropriate care in a culturally and ethnically sensitive manner.

- Engages in self-evaluation of practice on a regular basis, identifying areas of strength, as well as areas in which professional development would be beneficial.

- Obtains informal feedback regarding her or his own practice from healthcare consumers with IDD, family/legal guardians, peers, professional colleagues, and others, including direct care support professionals.

- Participates in systematic peer review as appropriate.

- Takes action to achieve goals identified during the evaluation process.

- Provides the evidence for practice decisions and actions as part of the informal and formal evaluation processes.

- Interacts with peers and colleagues to enhance her or his own professional nursing practice or role performance.

- Provides peers with formal or informal constructive feedback regarding their practice or role performance.

ADDITIONAL COMPETENCIES FOR THE APRN WHO SPECIALIZES IN IDD

The advanced practice registered nurse:

- Engages in a formal process seeking feedback regarding her or his own practice from healthcare consumers, peers, professional colleagues, and others, including direct care support professionals.

Standard 15. Resource Utilization

The registered nurse specializing in IDD utilizes appropriate resources to plan and provide nursing services that are safe, effective, and financially responsible to healthcare consumers with IDD.

COMPETENCIES

The registered nurse:

- Assesses healthcare consumer care needs and the resources available to achieve desired outcomes.

- Identifies resource allocation for the needs of the healthcare consumer with IDD, desired outcome, complexity of the strategy to meet the needs, and the potential for harm if needs are not addressed.

- Delegates elements of care to appropriate healthcare workers in accordance with any applicable legal or policy parameters or principles.

- Identifies the evidence when evaluating resources.

- Advocates for resources, including technology, that enhance nursing practice.

- Modifies practice when necessary to promote positive interaction between healthcare consumers with IDD, care providers, and technology.

- Assists the healthcare consumer with IDD and family/legal guardians in identifying and securing appropriate services to address needs across the healthcare continuum.

- Assists the healthcare consumer with IDD and family/legal guardians in factoring costs, risks, and benefits in decisions about treatment and care.

- Applies innovative solutions and strategies to obtain appropriate resources.

- Utilizes organizational resources to ensure a work environment that is conducive to completing the identified plan and outcomes.

■ Designs evaluation methods that measure safety and effectiveness of interventions and outcomes.

■ Promotes activities that assist others, as appropriate, in becoming informed about costs, risks, and benefits of care, or of the plan and solution.

ADDITIONAL COMPETENCIES FOR THE APRN WHO SPECIALIZES IN IDD

■ The advanced practice registered nurse:

■ Utilizes organizational and community resources to formulate inter-professional plans of care.

■ Formulates innovative solutions for healthcare consumer care that utilize resources effectively and maintain quality.

■ Designs evaluation strategies that demonstrate cost-effectiveness, cost benefit, and efficiency factors associated with nursing practice.

Standard 16. Environmental Health

The registered nurse specializing in IDD nursing practices in an environmentally safe and healthy manner.

COMPETENCIES

The registered nurse:

- Attains knowledge of environmental health concepts, such as implementation of environmental health strategies.

- Promotes a practice environment that reduces environmental health risks for workers and healthcare consumers with IDD.

- Assesses the practice environment for factors such as sound, odor, noise, and light that threaten health.

- Advocates for the judicious and appropriate use of products in health care.

- Communicates environmental health risks and exposure reduction strategies to healthcare consumers with IDD, families/legal guardians, colleagues, and communities.

- Utilizes scientific evidence to determine if a product or treatment is an environmental threat.

- Participates in strategies to promote healthy communities.

- Identifies developmental and behavioral characteristics that predispose healthcare consumers with IDD to increased risk of exposure to environmental hazards and risks.

- Carefully assesses the home, school, and/or work environments of healthcare consumers with IDD for potential threat of exposure to environmental hazards and risks.

- Uses knowledge of chronic health disorders and IDD to distinguish between signs and symptoms associated with disorders and disabilities and signs and symptoms associated with harmful environmental exposures.

■ Develops strategies to prevent and/or minimize environmental health risks for healthcare consumers with IDD.

ADDITIONAL COMPETENCIES FOR THE APRN WHO SPECIALIZES IN IDD

The advanced practice registered nurse:

■ Creates partnerships that promote sustainable environmental health policies and conditions.

■ Analyzes the impact of social, political, and economic influences on the environment and human health risk exposures.

■ Critically evaluates the manner in which environmental health issues are presented by the popular media.

■ Advocates for implementation of environmental principles for nursing practice.

■ Supports nurses in advocating for and implementing environmental principles in nursing practice.

Glossary

Advanced practice registered nurse (APRN). A nurse who has completed an accredited graduate-level education program preparing her or him for the role of certified nurse practitioner, certified registered nurse anesthetist, certified nurse-midwife, or clinical nurse specialist; has passed a national certification examination that measures the APRN role and population-focused competencies; maintains continued competence as evidenced by recertification; and is licensed to practice as an APRN (adapted from APRN Joint Dialogue Group, 2008).

Assessment. A systematic, dynamic process by which the registered nurse, through interaction with the patient, family/legal guardians, groups, communities, populations, and healthcare providers, collects and analyzes data. Assessment may include the following dimensions: physical, psychological, sociocultural, spiritual, cognitive, functional abilities, developmental, economic, and lifestyle.

Autonomy. The capacity of a nurse to determine her or his own actions through independent choice, including demonstration of competence, within the full scope of nursing practice.

Caregiver. A person who provides direct care for another, such as a child, dependent adult, the disabled, or the chronically ill.

Code of ethics (nursing). A list of provisions that makes explicit the primary goals, values, and obligations of the nursing profession and expresses its values, duties, and commitments to the society of which it is a part. In the United States, nurses abide by and adhere to *Code of Ethics for Nurses with Interpretive Statements* (ANA, 2001).

Collaborative care. Care based on interprofessional problem-solving in which there is respect for the perspectives, abilities, knowledge, and experiences of each person who is involved in making decisions that affect a healthcare consumer's health, education, and/or vocational goals and programs.

Competency. An expected and measurable level of nursing performance that integrates knowledge, skills, abilities, and judgment, based on established scientific knowledge and expectations for nursing practice.

Comprehensive care. Care that integrates health (primary, secondary, and tertiary levels) and social/family/legal guardian support programs with educational or vocational services.

Continuity of care. An interprofessional process that includes healthcare consumers, families/legal guardians, and other stakeholders in the development of a coordinated plan of care. This process facilitates the healthcare consumer's transition between settings and healthcare providers, based on changing needs and available resources.

Coordinated care. Care that facilitates access to needed resources and services and promotes continuity of care among multiple providers and diverse service systems. Work is done collaboratively with the healthcare consumer and/or family/legal guardians to achieve mutually agreed-upon goals. Timeliness, appropriateness, and completeness of care are central to this concept.

Cultural competence. Care that respects, honors, and incorporates beliefs, norms, attitudes, and life practices of healthcare consumers and their families/legal guardians congruent with their values and practices.

Delegation. The transfer of responsibility for the performance of a task from one individual to another while retaining accountability for the outcome. Example: The RN, in delegating a task to unlicensed assistive personnel, transfers the responsibility for performance of the task but retains professional accountability for the overall care.

Developmentally appropriate. Care focused on the unique needs of healthcare consumers to promote developmental skills and independence congruent with the healthcare consumer's present functional abilities rather than chronological age.

Developmental screening. Generally assessing a person's global or specific domains of development for evidence of developmental deviation. The results of screening are not diagnostic; if the results reveal a possibility of delay, they must be repeated within a short period of time. If developmental delay is suspected after the repeated screening, the person should be referred for diagnosis and appropriate treatment and intervention.

Diagnosis. A clinical judgment about the healthcare consumer's response to actual or potential health conditions or needs. The diagnosis provides the basis for development of a plan to achieve expected outcomes. Registered nurses use nursing and medical diagnoses depending upon educational and clinical preparation and legal authority.

Diagnostic overshadowing. Assigning a mental health diagnosis to a person with IDD because the person has IDD. Example: An adolescent with Down syndrome is "feeling down" after a breakup with a boyfriend. The adolescent's provider diagnoses depression without any assessment other than the history.

Early intervention. The provision of health, social, and educational services in an interprofessional setting for children from birth to three years of age who are at risk for or who have IDD.

Environment. The surrounding context, milieu, conditions, or atmosphere in which a registered nurse practices.

Environmental health. Aspects of human health, including quality of life, that are determined by physical, chemical, biological, social, and psychological problems in the environment. Also refers to the theory and practice of assessing, correcting, controlling, and preventing those factors in the environment that can potentially adversely affect the health of present and future generations.

Evaluation. The process of determining the progress toward attainment of expected outcomes, including the effectiveness of care.

Evidence-based practice. A scholarly and systematic problem-solving paradigm that results in the delivery of high-quality health care.

Expected outcomes. End results that are measurable, desirable, and observable, and translate into observable behaviors or relate to policies, funding, and/or organizations.

Family. Family of origin or significant others, such as legal guardians, if identified by the healthcare consumer.

Family-centered care. Care to healthcare consumers in need of special services (e.g., therapies, rehabilitation, adaptive equipment) that is provided within the context of the healthcare consumer's family. The strengths, individuality, and diversity of each family/legal guardian is acknowledged and valued. The cornerstone of family-centered care is a partnership between the family/legal guardians and the professionals.

Health. An experience that is often expressed in terms of wellness and illness, and may occur in the presence or absence of disease or injury.

Healthcare consumer. The person, client, family, group, community, or population who is the focus of attention and to whom the registered nurse is providing services as sanctioned by the state regulatory bodies.

Healthcare providers. Individuals with special expertise who provide healthcare services or assistance to healthcare consumers with IDD. They may include nurses, physicians, psychologists, social workers, nutritionist/dietitians, and various therapists.

Illness. The subjective experience of discomfort.

Implementation. Activities such as teaching, monitoring, providing, counseling, delegating, and coordinating.

Inclusion. Integration of all persons, regardless of special needs and disabilities and/or the environment (e.g., school, community, etc.), with typical peers in the least restrictive setting. Innovative programs geared to the healthcare consumer's strengths and capabilities must be provided.

Individualized education plan (IEP). An annual educational program plan and goals that are jointly determined by the school teachers, therapists, school nurse, and parents of the school-aged child with IDD and members of their support system. The IEP includes all developmental and academic testing results, the child's health status, and the child's strengths and weaknesses, as well as transition plans. This plan may include vocational goals beginning at age 14.

Individualized family service plan (IFSP). An annual family service plan that includes goals and interventions for the entire family of a child, aged birth to three years, with or at risk for an IDD. The IFSP includes the child's strengths and weaknesses, the results of developmental testing in all areas of adaptive living, family needs, the identification of community resources, and transitional plans to the school setting. This plan is devised by the interprofessional team and the parents/legal guardians of the child with IDD and members of their support system.

Individualized plan for employment (IPE). An annual work or habilitation plan, usually completed for adults with IDD that includes goals and interventions as determined by the healthcare consumer, his or her family/legal guardians, and the interprofessional team at the healthcare consumer's place of employment and/or residence. The IPE includes all developmental, adaptive skill levels, habilitative training and skill levels, and the healthcare consumer's strengths and weaknesses, which are summarized in the plan.

Individualized transition plan (ITP). An annual transition plan, to begin when the adolescent with IDD becomes 14 to 16 years of age. Includes goals and interventions as determined by the healthcare consumer, his or her family/legal guardians, and the interprofessional team for the transition to adulthood. The ITP also includes the healthcare consumer's health, developmental, and adaptive skill levels, strengths and weaknesses, and goals for a successful transition into adulthood that incorporates all aspects of the healthcare consumer's life.

Information. Data that are interpreted, organized, or structured.

Interprofessional. Reliant on the overlapping knowledge, skills, and abilities of each professional team member, resulting in synergistic effects by which outcomes are enhanced and become more comprehensive than a simple aggregation of the individual efforts of the team members.

Interprofessional team. A group of professionals with varied and specialized backgrounds who work with the healthcare consumer and/or family/legal guardians to make decisions about all aspects of the life of the healthcare consumer with IDD, including health, education, and vocational needs. This planning should be person-centered. The membership of the interprofessional team should be determined by the type of expertise needed to meet the healthcare consumer's needs.

Least restrictive environment. The environment that offers the person with IDD the least amount of restriction in carrying out activities of daily living.

Medical home. Care that uses primary care providers to ensure the delivery of coordinated, comprehensive care.

Normalization. Providing a supportive environment for healthcare consumers with IDD to make decisions regarding activities of daily living and to live as close as possible to the norms and patterns in the mainstream of the society in which they reside. If this is not possible, then supporting the family/legal guardians who care for the healthcare consumer with IDD.

Nursing. The protection, promotion, and optimization of health and abilities; prevention of illness and injury; alleviation of suffering through the diagnosis and treatment of human response; and advocacy in the care of individuals, families/legal guardians, communities, and populations.

Nursing practice. The collective professional activities of nurses, characterized by the interrelations of human responses, theory application, nursing actions, and outcomes.

Nursing process. A critical thinking model used by nurses that comprises the integration of the singular, concurrent actions of these six components: assessment, diagnosis, identification of outcomes, planning, implementation, and evaluation.

Patient. *See* Healthcare consumer.

Peer review. A collegial, systematic, and periodic process by which registered nurses are held accountable for practice and that fosters the refinement of a nurse's knowledge, skills, and decision-making at all levels and in all areas of practice.

Person-centered care. Care that is focused on the wishes of the healthcare consumer with IDD after the healthcare consumer (and the healthcare consumer's family/legal guardians) is fully informed of the knowledge and options available in regard to his or her care.

Plan. A comprehensive outline of the components that must be addressed to attain expected outcomes.

Quality. The degree to which health services for patients, families/legal guardians, groups, communities, or populations increase the likelihood of desired outcomes and are consistent with current professional knowledge.

Registered nurse (RN). An individual registered or licensed by a state, commonwealth, territory, government, or other regulatory body to practice as a registered nurse.

Scope of Nursing Practice. The description of the *who, what, where, when, why,* and *how* of nursing practice that addresses the range of nursing practice activities common to all registered nurses. When considered in conjunction with *Standards of Professional Nursing Practice* and *Code of Ethics for Nurses*, comprehensively describes the competent level of nursing common to all registered nurses.

Standards. Authoritative statements defined and promoted by the profession by which the quality of practice, service, or education can be evaluated.

Standards of Practice. Describe a competent level of nursing care as demonstrated by the nursing process. *See also* Nursing process.

Standards of Professional Nursing Practice. Authoritative statements of the duties that all registered nurses, regardless of role, population, or specialty, are expected to perform competently.

Standards of Professional Performance. Describe a competent level of behavior in the professional role.

References and Bibliography

Aggen, R. L., DeGennaro, M. D., Fox, L., Hahn, J. E., Logan, B. A., & VonFumetti, L. (1995). *Standards of developmental disabilities nursing practice.* Eugene, OR: Developmental Disabilities Nurses Association.

Aggen, R. L., & Moore, N. J. (1984). *Standards of nursing practice in mental retardation/developmental disabilities.* Albany, NY: New York State Office of Mental Retardation and Developmental Disabilities.

Aiken, L. H., Clarke, S. P., Sloan, D. M., Lake, E. T., & Cheney, T. (2008). Effects of hospital care environment in patient mortality and nurse outcomes. *Journal of Nursing Administration, 38,* 223–229.

American Association of Colleges of Nursing (AACN). (2004). *AACN position statement on the practice doctorate in nursing. October 2004.* Washington, DC: Author.

American Association of Colleges of Nursing (AACN). (2008). *The essentials of baccalaureate education for professional nursing practice.* Washington, DC: Author.

American Association of Critical Care Nurses. (2005). *AACN standards for establishing and maintaining healthy work environments.* Mission Viejo, CA: Author.

American Association on Intellectual and Developmental Disabilities & ARC of the United States. (2008). *Individual supports: Position statement.* Retrieved from http://www.aaidd.org/content_153.cfm?navID=39

American Nurses Association Consensus Committee. (1993). *National standards of nursing practice for early intervention services.* Lexington, KY: University of Kentucky, College of Nursing.

American Nurses Association Consensus Committee. (1994). *Standards of nursing practice for the care of children and adolescents with special health and developmental needs.* Lexington, KY: University of Kentucky, College of Nursing.

American Nurses Association (ANA). (2001). *Code of Ethics for Nurses with interpretive statements.* Washington, DC: American Nurses Publishing.

American Nurses Association (ANA). (2007a). *Principles of environmental health for nursing practice.* Silver Spring, MD: Nursesbooks.org.

American Nurses Association (ANA). (2007b). *Public health nursing: Scope and standards of practice* (2nd ed.). Silver Spring, MD: Nursesbooks.org.

American Nurses Association (ANA). (2008). *Professional role competence: ANA position statement.* Silver Spring, MD: Nursesbooks.org.

American Nurses Association (ANA). (2010a). *Nursing: Scope and standards of practice* (2nd ed.). Silver Spring, MD: Nursesbooks.org.

American Nurses Association (ANA). (2010b). *Nursing's social policy statement: The essence of the profession* (3rd ed.). Silver Spring, MD: Nursesbooks.org.

American Nurses Association & Nursing Division of the American Association on Mental Retardation. (2004). *Intellectual and developmental disabilities nursing: Scope and standards of practice.* Silver Spring, MD: Nursesbooks.org.

American Nurses Credentialing Center (ANCC). (2008). *A new model for ANCC's Magnet Recognition Program.* Silver Spring, MD: Author.

American Psychiatric Nurses Association, International Society of Psychiatric-Mental Health Nurses, & American Nurses Association. (2007). *Psychiatric-mental health nursing: Scope and standards of practice.* Silver Spring, MD: Nursesbooks.org.

APRN Joint Dialogue Group. (2008, July 7). *Consensus model for APRN regulation: Licensure, accreditation, certification & education.* Retrieved from http://www.nursingworld.org/ConsensusModelforAPRN

ARC of the United States & American Association on Intellectual and Developmental Disabilities. (2008a). *Health, mental health, vision, and dental care: Position statement.* Retrieved from http://www.aaidd.org /content_151.cfm?navID=37

ARC of the United States & American Association on Intellectual and Developmental Disabilities. (2008b). *Self-determination: Position statement.* Retrieved from http://www.aaidd.org/content_163 .cfm?navID=49

Austin, J., Challela, M., Huber, C., Sciarillo, W., & Stade, C. (1987). *Standards for the clinical advanced practice registered nurse in developmental disabilities/handicapping conditions.* Washington, DC: American Association of University Affiliated Programs.

Barclay, A., Goulet, L. R., Holtgrewe, M. M., & Sharp, A. R. (1962). Parental evaluations of clinical services for retarded children. *American Journal on Mental Deficiency, 67,* 231–237.

Barnard, K. E. (1966). Symposium on mental retardation. *Nursing Clinics of North America, 1*(4), 629–630.

Barnard, K. E. (1968). Teaching the retarded child is a family affair. *American Journal of Nursing, 68,* 305–311.

Benner, P. (1984). *From novice to expert: Excellence and power in clinical nursing practice.* Menlo Park, CA: Addison-Wesley.

Board of Higher Education & Massachusetts Organization of Nurse Executives (BHE/MONE). (2006). *Creativity and connections: Building the framework for the future of nursing education. Report from the Invitational Working Session, March 23-24, 2006.* Burlington, MA: MONE. Retrieved from http://www.mass.edu/currentinit /documents/NursingCreativityAndConnections.pdf

Braddock, D., Hemp, R., Rizzolo, M. C., Haffer, L., Tanis, E. S., & Wu, J. (2011). *The state of the states in developmental disabilities: 2008.* Washington, DC: American Association on Intellectual and Developmental Disabilities.

Bureau of Labor Statistics. (May 17, 2011). *Occupational employment and news release.* Retrieved from http://www.bls.gov/news.release/ocwage.htm

Committee on Disability in America, Field, M. J., & Jette, A. M. (2007). *The future of disability in America.* Washington, DC: National Academy Press.

Cowan, D. T., Norman, I., & Coopamah, V. P. (2007). Competence in nursing practice: A controversial concept—A focused review of literature. *Accident & Emergency Nursing, 15,* 20–26.

Devine, P. (1983). Mental retardation: An early subspecialty in psychiatric nursing. *Journal of Psychiatric Nursing & Mental Health Services, 21,* 21–30.

Dix, D. (1847). *The appeal of Dorothy Dix to Illinois General Assembly for better treatment of the insane.* Springfield, IL.

Dix, D. L. (1976). Memorial to the legislature of Massachusetts, 1843. In M. Rosen, G. R. Clark, & M. S. Kivitz (Eds.). *The history of mental retardation: Collected papers* (Vol. 1, pp. 1–30). Baltimore, MD: University Park Press.

Gallagher-Lepak, S., & Kubsch, S. (2009). Transpersonal caring: A nursing practice guideline. *Holistic Nursing Practice, 23,* 171–182.

Hagerty, B. M. K., Lynch-Sauer, K., Patusky, K. L., & Bouwseman, M. (1993). An emerging theory of human relatedness. *Image, 25,* 291–296.

Haynes, U. (1968). *Guidelines for nursing standards in residential centers for the mentally retarded.* Washington, DC: United Cerebral Palsy Association.

Haynes, U. (1974). *Overview of the National Collaborative Infant Project.* Washington, DC: United Cerebral Palsy Association.

Igoe, J. B., Green, P., Heim, H., Licata, M., MacDonough, G. P., & McHugh, B. A. (1980). *School nurses working with handicapped children.* Kansas

City, MO: American Nurses Association.

Institute of Medicine (IOM). (1999). *To err is human: Building a safer health system.* Washington, DC: National Academies Press.

Institute of Medicine (IOM). (2001). *Crossing the quality chasm: A new health system for the 21st century.* Washington, DC: National Academies Press.

Institute of Medicine (IOM). (2003). *Health professions education: A bridge to quality.* Washington, DC: National Academies Press.

Institute of Medicine (IOM). (2004). *Keeping patients safe: Transforming the work environment of nurses.* Washington, DC: National Academies Press.

Institute of Medicine (IOM). (2010). *The future of nursing: Leading change, advancing health.* Washington, DC: National Academies Press.

International Society of Nurses in Genetics, Inc. (ISONG) & American Nurses Association. (1998). *Statement on the scope and standards of genetics clinical nursing practice.* Washington, DC: American Nurses Publishing.

International Society of Nurses in Genetics, Inc. (ISONG) & American Nurses Association. (2006). *Genetics-genomics nursing: Scope and standards of practice.* Silver Spring, MD: Nursesbooks.org.

Kearney, S. H. (2009). *Report of findings from the Post Entry Competence Study. NCSBN Research Brief. 29: June.* Retrieved from http://www.ncsbn.org/986.htm

Kelly, L. A., McHugh, M. D., & Aiken, L. H. (2011). Nurse outcomes in Magnet® and non-Magnet hospitals. *Journal of Nursing Administration, 41,* 428–433.

Lazarus, J. B., & Lee, N. G. (2006). Factoring consumers' perspectives into policy decisions for nursing competence. *Policy, Politics, & Nursing Practice, 7,* 195–207.

Leininger, M. M. (1988). Leininger's theory of nursing: Cultural care diversity and universality. *Nursing Science Quarterly, 1*(4), 152–160.

McMullan, M., Endacott, R., Gray, M., Jasper, M., Miller, C., Scholes, J., et al. (2003). Portfolios and assessment of competence: A review of the literature. *Journal of Advanced Nursing, 41*, 283–294.

McNelly, P. C. (1966, December). *Operation six-pack.* Paper presented at the Academy for Cerebral Palsy Meeting. New Orleans, LA (December 2-6).

Midwest Bioethics Center & University of Missouri-Kansas City Task Force on Health Care for Adults with Developmental Disabilities. (1996). Health care treatment decision-making guidelines for adults with developmental disabilities. *Bioethics Forum, 12*(3, Suppl.), 1–8.

Miller, J. A. (1979). *A history of nursing at Central Wisconsin Center for the developmentally disabled.* Unpublished manuscript, University of Illinois at Chicago.

National Association of School Nurses & American Nurses Association. (2011). *School nursing: Scope and standards of practice* (2nd ed.). Silver Spring, MD: Nursesbooks.org.

National Council of State Boards of Nursing (NCSBN). (2005). *Meeting the ongoing challenge of continued competence.* Chicago, IL: Author. http://www.ncsbn.org

Nehring, W. M. (1999). *A history of nursing in the field of mental retardation and developmental disabilities.* Washington, DC: American Association on Mental Retardation.

Nehring, W. M. (Ed.). (2005). *Core curriculum for specializing in intellectual and developmental disability: A resource for nurses and other health care professionals.* Boston, MA: Jones and Bartlett.

Nehring, W. M. (2010). Historical perspectives on emerging trends. In C. L. Betz & W. M. Nehring (Eds.), *Nursing care for individuals with intellectual and developmental disabilities: An integrated approach* (pp. 1–18). Baltimore, MD: Paul H. Brookes.

Nightingale, F. (1859). *Notes on nursing: What it is and what it is not.* London, UK: John W. Parker and Son.

Nursing Division of the American Association on Mental Retardation & American Nurses Association. (1998). *Statement on the scope and standards for the nurse who specializes in developmental disabilities and/ or mental retardation.* Washington, DC: American Nurses Publishing.

Papastavrou, E., Efstathiou, G., Acaroglu, R., Luz, M. D., Berg, A., Idvall, E., et al. (2011). A seven country comparison of nurses' perceptions of their professional practice environment. *Journal of Nursing Management.* doi:10.1111/j.1365-2834.2011.01289.x.

Pope, A. M., & Tarlov, A. R. (Eds.). (1991). *Disability in America: Toward a national agenda for prevention.* Washington, DC: National Academies Press.

Roth, S. P., & Morse, J. S. (Eds.). (1994). *A life-span approach to nursing care for individuals with developmental disabilities.* Baltimore, MD: Paul H. Brookes.

Roth, W. L. (1945). *The New York Hospital: A history of the psychiatric service 1771–1936.* New York, NY: Columbia University Press.

Russell, W. L. (1945). *The New York Hospital: A history of the psychiatric service 1771–1936.* New York, NY: Columbia University Press.

Schalock, R. L., Borthwick-Duffy, S. A., Bradley, V. J., Buntinx, W. H. E., Coulter, D. L., Craig, E. M., et al. (2010). *Intellectual disabilities: Definition, classification, and systems of supports* (11th ed.). Washington, DC: American Association on Intellectual and Developmental Disabilities.

Scott Tilley, D. D. (2008). Competency in nursing: A concept analysis. *Journal of Continuing Education in Nursing, 39*(2), 58–64.

Society of Pediatric Nurses, National Association of Pediatric Nurse Practitioners, & American Nurses Association. (2008). *Pediatric nursing: Scope and standards of practice.* Silver Spring, MD: Nursesbooks.org.

Styles, M. M., Schumann, M. J., Bickford, C. J., & White, K. (2008). *Specializing and credentialing in nursing revisited: Understanding the issues, advancing the profession.* Silver Spring, MD: American Nurses Association.

Sumner, G., & Spietz, A. (1994). *NCAST caregiver/parent-child interaction teaching manual.* Seattle, WA: NCAST Publications, University of Washington, School of Nursing.

Swanson, K. (1993). Empirical development of a middle-range theory of caring. *Nursing Research, 40*(3), 161–166.

U.S. Public Health Service. (2002). *Closing the gap: A national blueprint for improving the health of individuals with mental retardation.* (Report of the Surgeon General's Conference on Health Disparities and Mental Retardation.) Washington, DC: Author.

Watson, J. (1999). *Postmodern nursing and beyond.* Edinburgh, UK: Churchill Livingstone.

Watson, J. (2008). *The philosophy and science of caring.* Boulder, CO: University Press of Colorado.

Appendix A.

Intellectual and Developmental Disabilities Nursing: Scope and Standards of Practice (2004)

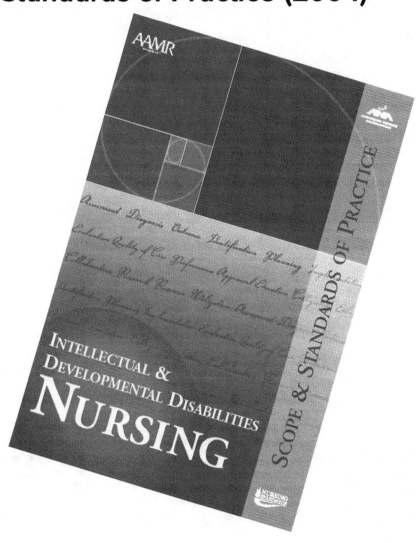

INTELLECTUAL AND DEVELOPMENTAL DISABILITIES NURSING:
SCOPE AND STANDARDS OF PRACTICE

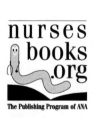

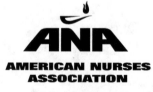

SILVER SPRING, MARYLAND
2004

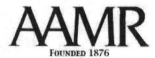

The content in this appendix is not current and is of historical significance only.

ACKNOWLEDGMENTS

The Nursing Division of the American Association on Mental Retardation and the American Nurses Association would like to personally thank those who contributed their valuable time and talents to this revised edition, *Intellectual and Developmental Disabilities Nursing: Scope and Standards of Practice.* In its original (1988) edition, the document was called *Statement on the Scope and Standards for the Nurse Who Specializes in Developmental Disabilities and/or Mental Retardation.*

The authors of the *Intellectual and Developmental Disabilities Nursing: Scope and Standards of Practice* include:

Wendy M. Nehring, RN, PhD, FAAN, FAAMR
Shirley P. Roth, RN, MSN, FAAMR
Deborah Natvig, RN, PhD
Cecily L. Betz, RN, PhD, FAAN
Teresa Savage, RN, PhD
Marilyn Krajicek, RN, EdD, FAAN

Special thanks are extended to Lee Barks, RN, MS, ARNP, and Sally Colatarci, RN, MS for their suggestions.

ANA Staff

Carol Bickford, PhD, RN,BC – Content Editor
Yvonne Humes, MSA
Winifred Carson-Smith, JD

The content in this appendix is not current and is of historical significance only.

CONTENTS

The content in this appendix is not current and is of historical significance only.

The content in this appendix is not current and is of historical significance only.

PREFACE

The American Nurses Association (ANA) has been the vanguard for nursing practice for more than a century. *Code of Ethics for Nurses with Interpretive Statements* (ANA 2001), *Nursing: Scope and Standards of Practice* (ANA 2004), and *Nursing's Social Policy Statement* (2nd ed.) (ANA 2003) are all documents that provide background for nursing standards. These documents are intended to provide the public with assurances of safe and competent nursing care. Along with these documents, specialty nursing organizations have worked with the ANA to publish specific standards of care and professional practice in their specialty.

This document, concerning the care of individuals with intellectual and developmental disabilities (hereafter referred to as I/DD), is a revision of *Statement on the Scope and Standards for the Nurse Who Specializes in Developmental Disabilities and/or Mental Retardation* (Nehring et al. 1998).

This new document has been revised to: (*i*) capture the changing practice of nursing in this specialty (i.e., encompassing all levels of education, all system levels of care from the individual to the system itself), (*ii*) emphasize the unique healthcare needs and characteristics of individuals of all ages with I/DD, and (*iii*) to incorporate the ANA standards mentioned above (ANA, 2004). It should also be used in conjunction with other standards of care and professional performance developed by other specialty nursing groups [e.g., *Scope and Standards of Pediatric Nursing Practice* (Society of Pediatric Nurses & ANA, 2003); *Statement on the Scope and Standards of Genetics Clinical Nursing Practice* (International Society of Nurses in Genetics, Inc. & ANA, 1998); *Scope and Standards of Public Health Nursing Practice* (ANA, 1999); *Scope and Standards of Psychiatric–Mental Health Nursing Practice* (American Psychiatric Nurses Association, International Society of Psychiatric–Mental Health Nurses, & ANA, 2000); and *Scope and Standards of Professional School Nursing Practice* (National Association of School Nurses & ANA, 2001).

The content in this appendix is not current and is of historical significance only.

In addition, adolescents and adults with I/DD and their families collaborate with healthcare professionals in making person-centered decisions about their health care. This self-advocacy has arisen in tandem with an evolving healthcare system that may or may not optimize healthcare options for all people. Therefore, in response to these changes, individuals of all ages with I/DD and their families should be assured of safe and effective nursing care. This document describes this care.

The content in this appendix is not current and is of historical significance only.

STANDARDS OF INTELLECTUAL AND DEVELOPMENTAL DISABILITIES (I/DD) NURSING PRACTICE: STANDARDS OF PRACTICE

STANDARD 1. ASSESSMENT
The registered nurse who specializes in I/DD collects comprehensive data pertinent to the patient's health or the situation.

STANDARD 2. DIAGNOSIS
The registered nurse who specializes in I/DD analyzes the assessment data to determine the diagnoses or issues.

STANDARD 3. OUTCOMES IDENTIFICATION
The registered nurse who specializes in I/DD identifies expected outcomes for a plan to the patient or the situation.

STANDARD 4. PLANNING
The registered nurse who specializes in I/DD develops a plan that prescribes strategies and alternatives to attain expected outcomes.

STANDARD 5. IMPLEMENTATION
The registered nurse who specializes in I/DD implements the identified plan.

STANDARD 5A: COORDINATION OF CARE
The registered nurse who specializes in I/DD coordinates care delivery.

STANDARD 5B: HEALTH TEACHING AND HEALTH PROMOTION
The registered nurse who specializes in I/DD employs strategies to promote health and a safe environment.

STANDARD 5C: CONSULTATION
The registered nurse and the advanced practice registered nurse who specializes in I/DD provide consultation to influence the identified plan, enhance the abilities of others, and effect change.

STANDARD 5D: PRESCRIPTIVE AUTHORITY AND TREATMENT
The advanced practice registered nurse who specializes in I/DD uses prescriptive authority, procedures, referrals, treatments, and therapies in accordance with state and federal laws and regulations.

STANDARD 6: EVALUATION
The registered nurse who specializes in I/DD evaluates progress toward attainment of outcomes.

The content in this appendix is not current and is of historical significance only.

Standards of Intellectual and Developmental Disabilities (I/DD) Nursing Practice: Standards of Professional Performance

STANDARD 7. QUALITY OF PRACTICE

The registered nurse who specializes in I/DD systematically enhances the quality and effectiveness of nursing practice.

STANDARD 8. EDUCATION

The registered nurse who specializes in I/DD attains knowledge and competency that reflects current nursing practice.

STANDARD 9. PROFESSIONAL PRACTICE EVALUATION

The registered nurse who specializes in I/DD evaluates one's own nursing practice in relation to professional practice standards and guidelines, relevant statutes, rules, and regulations.

STANDARD 10. COLLEGIALITY

The registered nurse who specializes in I/DD interacts with and contributes to the professional development of peers and colleagues.

STANDARD 11. COLLABORATION

The registered nurse who specializes in I/DD collaborates with the individual with I/DD, family, and others in the conduct of nursing practice.

STANDARD 12. ETHICS

The registered nurse who specializes in I/DD integrates ethical provisions in all areas of practice.

STANDARD 13. RESEARCH

The registered nurse who specializes in I/DD integrates research findings into practice.

STANDARD 14. RESOURCE UTILIZATION

The registered nurse specializing in I/DD considers factors related to safety, effectiveness, cost, and impact on practice in the planning and delivery of nursing services to individuals with I/DD.

STANDARD 15. LEADERSHIP

The nurse who specializes in I/DD provides leadership in the professional practice setting and the profession.

Scope of Practice of Intellectual and Developmental Disabilities (I/DD) Nursing

Nurses who specialize in intellectual and developmental disabilities (I/DD) are unique in the population that they serve. Because this nursing specialty was primarily institutional until the late 1950s, and because of the stigma attached to this population, many nurses are not familiar with this nursing specialty. In fact, it was only recognized as such by the American Nurses Association (ANA) in 1997 (Nehring, 1999).

Unlike many nursing specialties, the scope of practice for nurses in I/DD extends across all levels of care, as well as all healthcare and many educational settings. Even though individuals with I/DD are present today in all communities and healthcare settings, they remain a vulnerable population. This is because they often need assistance to advocate for their needs and many healthcare professionals are not educated and skilled to care for their specific condition and developmental needs. Such health disparities were highlighted in the Surgeon General's report, *Closing the Gap: A National Blueprint to Improve the Health of Persons with Mental Retardation* (U.S. Public Health Service 2002). Working in an interdisciplinary context, nurses continue to strive to promote the importance of the discipline of nursing in this specialty field and to provide specific health care at both the generalist and advanced practice level.

Definition of Nursing in I/DD

Intellectual and developmental disability refers to a wide variety of mental or physical conditions that interfere with the ability of an individual to function effectively at an expected developmental level. These conditions are frequently referred to as *developmental disabilities* or *mental retardation.* A *developmental disability* is:

> a severe chronic disability of an individual that (a) is attributable to mental or physical impairment or combination of mental and physical impairments; (b) is manifested before the individual attains the age of 22; (c) is likely to continue indefinitely; (d) re-

sults in substantial functional limitations in these following areas of major life activity: self-care, receptive and expressive living, and economic self-sufficiency; and (e) reflects the individual's need for a combination and sequence of special, interdisciplinary, or generic services, individualized support, or other forms of assistance that are of lifelong or extended duration and are individually planned and coordinated. (Developmental Disabilities Assistance and Bill of Rights Act of 2000)

The definition of *mental retardation* is:

a disability characterized by significant limitations both in intellectual functioning and in adaptive behavior as expressed in conceptual, social, and practical adaptive skills. This disability originates before age 18. The following five assumptions are essential to the application of this definition: (a) limitations in present functioning must be considered within the context of community environments typical of the individual's age peers and culture; (b) valid assessment considers cultural and linguistic diversity as well as differences in communication, sensory, motor, and behavioral factors; (c) within an individual, limitations often coexist with strengths; (d) an important purpose of describing limitations is to develop a profile of needed supports; and (e) with appropriate personalized supports over a sustained period, the life functioning of the person with mental retardation generally will improve. (Luckasson et al. 2002, 1).

Nurses who specialize in the care of persons of all ages with I/DD care for persons with these conditions. These conditions may be organic and nonorganic or social in nature.

It is important to clarify that I/DD is different from chronic conditions or illness and disabilities in general. *Chronic conditions* can simply mean any condition that persists over a long period. Although I/DD exists across time, the definition is more specific. This is also true for *disabilities,* a general term that refers to any condition that limits activities of daily living. Again, I/DD may limit activities of daily living, but the conditions require more specific understanding of epidemiology, etiology, diagnosis, treatment and management, follow-up, and nursing implications.

Another term often used is *children with special healthcare needs.* Children with I/DD often have special healthcare needs, but this may not be a consistent problem. For example, a child with Down syndrome may have special needs, but they may not always concern their health at any given time.

It is important, as new terminology is used, to identify and describe particular conditions (e.g., pervasive developmental disabilities and special-needs child), so that nurses do not lose sight of the knowledge and skills needed to care for persons with I/DD, regardless of the diagnosis. Although the terms to describe I/DD may overlap (i.e., developmental disabilities and special healthcare needs in the child with cerebral palsy), the definitions for developmental disabilities and mental retardation are used in federal legislation and must be understood by nurses until these definitions are altered.

Evolution of Nursing Practice in I/DD

Early education for nurses who specialized in the care of persons, of any age, with I/DD occurred both in general nursing hospital schools and in asylums and institutions. Until the early twentieth century, persons with I/DD were diagnosed as having mental illness, and their care took place in settings where persons with all forms of mental illness were housed. It was not until after World War I, when a better understanding of mental illness developed, that the care of persons with I/DD was more specifically detailed. Terminology at this time included *idiocy* and *imbecile.* In the early 1960s, President Kennedy brought needed attention to the living conditions of persons of all ages with I/DD, then called *mental retardation.* New legislation was introduced and funding became available for the first time for this population. Large institutional settings remained the primary place of residence for persons of all ages with I/DD until the late 1960s. It was the social norm to place newborns and children with known conditions resulting in I/DD in institutions as soon as possible so as not to burden the families, either financially or through social stigma.

After public attention was focused on the custodial and often inhumane care of persons with I/DD in the early 1970s, radical changes took place. Many individuals with I/DD were moved back to their homes or

The content in this appendix is not current and is of historical significance only.

to newly formed community settings such as group homes, semi-independent living arrangements (SILAs), and smaller, congregate settings (e.g., 16-beds). The transition from institutional to community living varies state by state. Today, newborns with I/DD are no longer placed in institutions. Most individuals with I/DD live with their families in the community. Others live in small group community settings; only the most severely affected individuals who require substantial medical care remain in larger, developmental centers (Nehring, 1999).

Nursing care has also evolved. Early documentation about nursing care was written by physicians or nurses who cared for persons with both I/DD and mental illness. Specific literature on the nursing care of persons with I/DD written by nurses first appeared with any frequency in the 1950s. At that time, nurses in institutional settings did little more than record vital signs and occasional patient weights and give medications. Public health nurses also provided care for children with I/DD who remained at home. However, parents were often encouraged to enroll their children in institutions by the time they reached school age. The first national meeting for nurses specializing in the care of children with I/DD was sponsored by the Children's Bureau in 1958 (Nehring, 1999).

In the 1960s, nursing care in the institution resembled that of nursing care provided in hospitals. Subsequently, the role of the nurse expanded to include education and research. Clinical advanced practice registered nurses were employed by some institutions and post-baccalaureate and graduate programs emerged to provide education designed especially for the care of children and adolescents with I/DD in universities across the country. Interdisciplinary faculty (including nurses) at University-Affiliated Programs and Facilities (UAPs or UAFs) established by President Kennedy, offered education to future specialists in this field (including nurses), conducted research on topics related to mental retardation, and provided health and social services to individuals with I/DD and their families.

Also during this time, nurses began to write more prolifically about the care of children with conditions resulting in I/DD. Some of the resulting books and articles are now classics, especially for public health nurses. Developmental diagnostic clinics were established across the country to identify and refer children for developmental and health care when appropriate. Nursing consultants who specialized in this field were hired by the Children's Bureau; Division of Neurological Diseases and Stroke, U.S. Public Health Service; Mental Retardation Division, Department of Health, Education, and Welfare; Association of Retarded Children; and the United Cerebral Palsy Associations, Inc. National meetings were convened for these nursing specialists and the first standards of nursing practice for this specialty emerged in 1968, *The Guidelines for Nursing Standards in Residential Centers for the Mentally Retarded* (Haynes, 1968; Nehring, 1999).

The 1970s brought about the first legislation mandating that all children with I/DD deserved a free and appropriate public education from 3 through 21 years of age. Advanced practice roles for nurses in this specialty continued to expand, including roles in schools and early intervention programs for the infant from birth to 3 years of age. Publications and regular national and regional meetings continued to be held throughout this decade. Special courses in this specialty also began to appear in nursing programs across the country (Nehring, 1999).

The term *developmental disabilities* was first introduced during the Nixon presidency to describe conditions similar to those defined as mental retardation but that differed slightly. Interdisciplinary care was the norm in the 1980s, when all disciplines worked together with the individuals with I/DD and their family members in assessing and planning care in a variety of settings (Nehring, 1999). In 1980, the American Nurses Association published *School Nurses Working with Handicapped Children* (Igoe, Green, Heim, Licata, MacDonough, and McHugh, 1980). In the 1980s, two sets of standards of nursing practice for nurses specializing in this field emerged: *Standards of Nursing Practice in Mental Retardation/Developmental Disabilities* (Aggen and Moore, 1984) and *Standards for the Clinical Advanced Practice Registered Nurse in Developmental Disabilities/Handicapping Conditions* (Austin, Challela, Huber, Sciarillo, and Stade, 1987).

Emphasis on the adult with I/DD emerged in the nursing literature in the 1990s. An examination of the individual with I/DD across the lifespan was first highlighted in *A Life-Span Approach to Nursing Care for Individuals with Developmental Disabilities* (Roth and Morse, 1994). Nursing standards for this field were also revised: *Standards of Developmental Disabilities Nursing Practice* (Aggen et al., 1995) and *Statement on the Scope and*

The content in this appendix is not current and is of historical significance only.

Standards for the Nurse Who Specializes in Developmental Disabilities and/ or Mental Retardation (Nehring et al., 1998). Other related standards of nursing practice in early intervention (Consensus Committee, 1993), care of children and adolescents with special health and developmental needs (Consensus Committee, 1994), and genetics (International Society of Nurses in Genetics, Inc. and ANA, 1998) were written.

In the first years of the twenty-first century, a greater effort in providing educational materials for nursing students and nurses in practice who care for persons of all ages with I/DD has emerged. The Nursing Division of the American Association on Mental Retardation and the Developmental Disabilities Nurses Association have been developing separate, but complementary, projects that will provide a core curriculum for nurses and other health professionals and Internet materials, respectively.

This specialty field of nursing has changed greatly from its early years. As the healthcare system continues to evolve, so will the nursing care of persons of all ages with I/DD. Such care continues to occur in a variety of settings and at both the professional registered nurse and advanced practice registered nurse levels. Continued publications and research into such nursing care are needed as well as additional didactic and clinical content materials for nursing students.

Integrating the Science and Art of Nursing in I/DD

Like the discipline of nursing in general, the nursing specialty of I/DD is based on the nursing process whereby critical thinking is used to assess and identify health problems, determine desired outcomes, plan and act, and evaluate the nursing care. Nursing care in this specialty is defined by the standards of nursing practice and professional performance for nurses who specialize in I/DD (see Figure 1 on the following page).

The art of nursing in this specialty is also dynamic and encompasses a holistic approach in providing care. For example, the person with I/DD may have difficulty communicating or be unable to communicate. Thus, the nurse must have skills to understand and interpret the signs or signals that the individual with I/DD uses to communicate their wants and desires.

The content in this appendix is not current and is of historical significance only.

Figure 1. The Phenomena of Concern for Nurses Who Specialize in I/DD

Individuals
- Unique anatomical, physiological, and psychological differences depending on diagnosis (e.g., genetic syndromes, congenital defects, physical deformities).
- Developmental interventions based on developmental or functional rather than chronological age.
- Prevention of secondary impairments.
- Adequate and appropriate primary health care and immunizations based on chronological age.
- Appropriate management of acute and chronic illnesses.
- Consistent collaboration with the individual regarding management of health care (person-centered care).
- Appropriate healthcare teaching at the individual's developmental level.
- Holistic management of psychosocial concerns; i.e. caring for the whole person.
- Developing, implementing, and evaluating the Individualized Family Service Plan (IFSP), Individualized Education Plan (IEP), Individualized Health Plan (IHP), Individualized Plan for Employment (IPE), or Individualized Transition Plan (ITP) with the interdisciplinary team which includes the person with I/DD and their family members.
- Advocacy.
- Legal issues or concerns.
- Respect for cultural, religious, and socioeconomic differences.

Family
- Family-centered approach that is respectful of cultural, religious, and socioeconomic differences.
- Continuous collaboration with family members regarding management of health care.
- Advocacy.
- Sensitivity to family concerns that support quality of life for persons with I/DD.

Community
- Case management across the person's lifespan.
- Keeping abreast of advances in nursing and the other disciplines involved in the care of persons with I/DD.
- Economic and political changes and their influence on financial status of the family (e.g., changes in SSI policy).
- Keeping abreast of political and policy changes and being able to translate these changes to the individual and their family.

Ethical issues are very important to understanding and caring for the person with I/DD. In general, people with I/DD should no longer be seen as vulnerable and dependent. They should be viewed as self-advocates who may need some level of support to function in society. The medical model of disability views the disability as a problem within the person, to be cured or ameliorated by professionals of medicine or other social institutions, and views the disability negatively (Williams, 2001, 125-7). By contrast, the social model of disability views disability as a socially constructed phenomenon in which an impairment becomes a disability when physical, social, or attitudinal barriers prevent the per-

The content in this appendix is not current and is of historical significance only.

son from attaining goals. The disability is seen as neutral and not from a value-laden perspective. The person may require accommodation to function and attain goals (Asch 2001, 300).

The nurse respects and facilitates the person's autonomy and decision-making capacity. Even individuals with guardians should be involved in their healthcare decisions to the extent of their ability to participate in decision-making. Nurses recognize that the current health-care system has constraints, and they must advocate and work within the limits to allow the individual with I/DD to have choices. However, the trend toward limited guardianship rather than plenary guardianship indicates that the person with I/DD is approaching equality in society.

With increasing medical and assistive technology, gains have been made in health and functional status for people with I/DD. Technology has also posed threats, as bioethicists have challenged the use of technology for persons with "severe" I/DD (Nerney, 2000, 15–20). Futility policies for persons with significant cognitive impairment have been instituted (Burling 2002), and medical decision-making guidelines for withholding resuscitation of infants who are extremely premature or born with congenital anomalies have been proposed (Colorado Collective for Medical Decisions, 1999). These activities display a bias against people with I/DD, even those who are at risk for I/DD. Nurses should advocate for a careful evaluation of the benefits and burdens of a proposed treatment for a person with I/DD (or at risk for I/DD) and not accept a categorical denial of treatment based on another's estimation of the quality of life of the person with or at risk for I/DD.

The Human Genome Project also poses gains and threats to people with I/DD. Sometime in the future, the basis for I/DD may be identified and eventually "treated" with gene therapy. If this technology evolves, there may be social pressure to submit to the treatment to ameliorate or eliminate the disability, showing less tolerance for the spectrum of human difference. Already there is an assumption if a prenatal disability is detected, the mother (or parents) will elect to terminate the pregnancy. Nurses respect the autonomous decisions of the mother, but also grant that the mother's decision may be influenced by the treatment of people with I/DD within society and its lack of tolerance for difference.

As stated in *Nursing's Social Policy Statement* (2003), "Human experience is contextually and culturally defined" (2). Nurses should be mindful of the experience of people with I/DD in society as one of oppression and denial of equality. Health services such as routine gynecological care, mammograms, and preventative and therapeutic dental services should be accessible to people with I/DD. There should be a balance between *undertreatment*—the limitations of treatment based on the I/DD diagnosis—and *overtreatment*—the unwillingness to recognize when treatment is no longer beneficial. Nurses may have advocacy and educator roles in the decision-making process with the person, if capable, the family, if appropriate, and others involved in the person's care.

In addition to the significant ethical concerns and issues, nurses must be knowledgeable of psychological, social, economic, cultural, and legal issues. Nurses must grasp the interdisciplinary nature of health care in this field and be prepared to provide case management of individuals with I/DD. Nurses at any level of practice must also be active in nursing and specialty organizations at local, regional, national, or international levels. Nursing leadership is important in these organizations at all levels, as well as in the communities.

Professional Registered Nurses Who Specialize in I/DD

In the United States, professional registered nurses receive their education through three routes: associate degree (2 years), diploma (3 years), or baccalaureate degree (4 years). This education prepares the professional registered nurse to practice in a variety of specialties and settings. In these educational programs, the nursing student receives didactic and clinical experiences in I/DD, but does not specialize in this area as part of their pre-licensure program.

All nurses will care for an individual with I/DD at some time in their careers. Each person with I/DD is a person first, just like everyone else, and their healthcare needs are unique to that individual. It is important that nurses recognize that a person with I/DD:

- is not ill based on their diagnosis of a I/DD,

- does not necessarily have all of the secondary conditions identified as common to their diagnosis (e.g., a person with spina bifida does not always have hydrocephaly), and

The content in this appendix is not current and is of historical significance only.

- experiences many of the same life events (e.g., graduation, first job, etc.) and has the same feelings that all of us do.

It is important to avoid diagnostic overshadowing (attributing a health problem to the person's diagnosis of I/DD; e.g., an adolescent with Down syndrome who is depressed because they broke up with their girlfriend is thought to be depressed because they have Down syndrome). In most pre-license nursing programs, the attention to the care of persons with I/DD is small, but nurses practicing as registered nurses must be able to provide holistic care to this population. Many books, articles, videos, and Internet sites are available to assist in this learning. The registered nurse may also want to consult with a nurse specialist in this field.

The professional registered nurse who specializes in I/DD provides care to individuals, families, and groups in a wide range of care settings with an understanding of the concepts and strategies of nursing practice in this area. The professional registered nurse participates in individual and family assessment and in the planning, implementation, and evaluation of their health and health services. The professional registered nurse may serve as a case manager as part of an interdisciplinary team with individuals with I/DD who have less complex needs if an advanced practice registered nurse is not available. The professional registered nurse collaborates and consults with the advanced practice registered nurse in I/DD as a resource. If no advanced practice registered nurse is available in the practice setting, advanced practice registered nurses who can serve as consultants may be available through the Nursing Division of the American Association on Mental Retardation or through University Centers of Excellence in Developmental Disabilities (UCEDDs, formerly UAPs or UAFs).

Certification as a certified developmental disabilities nurse is available from the Developmental Disabilities Nurses Association. One requirement for taking the certification examination is 4000 hours experience working as a professional registered nurse in a setting with individuals with I/DD in the past 5 years.

Advanced Practice Registered Nurses Who Specialize in I/DD

The majority of advanced practice professional nurses will care for persons with I/DD in their careers. The nurse practitioner may encounter

The content in this appendix is not current and is of historical significance only.

the pregnant woman with I/DD, the birth of a child with I/DD, the diagnosis of I/DD in a child, the care of the child with I/DD throughout childhood and adolescence to the transition to adulthood and adult health care, adult health services, psychiatric–mental health services, and finally, older adult services. The nurse practitioner may carry out these services in the clinic, hospital, school, home, or residential setting. The clinical nurse specialist, in any area of specialty, may encounter a person with I/DD in the hospital or clinic setting. The nurse midwife will most likely be involved someday in the birth of a child with I/DD or care for a woman with I/DD who is having a baby. The nurse anesthetist may also care for an individual with I/DD who is undergoing surgery.

As in pre-licensure nursing education, little attention is given to the healthcare needs of persons with I/DD in graduate nursing programs, unless the student chooses to specialize in this field. All nurses, regardless of educational preparation, must be prepared for the unique healthcare needs of persons with I/DD and always include the individual's family and additional support persons, if applicable, in all discussions of care. As stated, there are many resources available to nurses to enhance their knowledge and skills in this area, including consultation with master's and doctorally prepared nurse specialists.

It is recommended that the nurse who would like to specialize in I/DD in either their master's or doctoral program needs to attend a nursing program that is located at the same university where a UCEDD is located. Fellowships are usually available at UCEDDs for interdisciplinary education. The nursing master's student would be able to take interdisciplinary didactic courses at the UCEDD and participate in clinical practicums that involve individuals with I/DD and their families. The nursing doctoral student could also participate in the didactic interdisciplinary courses as cognates and plan and conduct their dissertation research with the assistance of the UCEDD faculty. If this is not possible, it is important for the nurse wishing to specialize in I/DD to inquire of the nursing faculty at the university that they would like to attend about how they could obtain needed interdisciplinary courses and clinical experiences. It would be very important that at least one nursing faculty be an expert in I/DD.

The content in this appendix is not current and is of historical significance only.

The master's or doctorally prepared nurse who specializes in I/DD is an advanced practice registered nurse or specialist who is capable of, and has the authority to perform, all of the functions of the professional registered nurse with a more independent and sophisticated conceptually grounded focus.

- The master's-prepared nurse in this specialty may be clinically employed in the role of clinical advanced practice registered nurse, nurse consultant, nurse practitioner, nurse educator, or nurse administrator.

- The doctorally prepared nurse in this specialty may function in a clinical, educational, administrative, consultative, or research role. In addition, the advanced practice registered nurse possesses substantial experience with individuals with I/DD, their families, and community resources; skill in the formulation and implementation of social policy and legislation affecting persons with I/DD; the ability to plan, implement, and evaluate programs designed to serve individuals with I/DD and their families; and their ability to conduct research.

These skills are based on knowledge of specific I/DD, including their epidemiology and demographics. The advanced practice registered nurse understands the use of technology for persons with I/DD as well as the impact of social, psychological, educational, cultural, and religious values on individuals, their families, and communities. The advanced practice registered nurse in I/DD must be knowledgeable about cost containment, legislation, and policy planning to provide preventive, supportive, and restorative care to individuals with I/DD across the lifespan in a wide variety of settings.

The advanced practice registered nurse is prepared to engage in interdisciplinary assessments, interventions, and teaching with an emphasis on individual- and family-centered services delivered within a community context. The advanced practice registered nurse is also able to serve as a case manager and interdisciplinary team leader, and to identify and develop a program of research relevant to the practice of nursing in I/DD. This document emphasizes the development and maintenance of skills necessary to promote positive health outcomes for the entire population of individuals with I/DD; it does not focus on a particular clinical diagnosis.

Settings for Nursing Practice in I/DD

Nursing in I/DD is the care of persons with I/DD and their families across a variety of healthcare, educational, and residential settings. These settings include large public and private agencies (such as hospitals, clinics, public health clinics, worksites, and schools), small community-based facilities, large regional developmental centers, foster homes, and biological homes. The nurse who practices in this specialty may serve in several capacities, including (a) clinician, (b) teacher, (c) interdisciplinary team member, (d) case manager, (e) advocate, (f) counselor, (g) consultant, (h) administrator, and (i) researcher (Nehring, 2003). Nurses who specialize in I/DD have a broad range of concerns in providing holistic care to individuals, families, and communities (see Figure 1).

Continued Commitment to the Nursing Specialty of I/DD

The nurse's practice in I/DD is both independent and collaborative. Under professional licensure, the nurse's independent responsibility is screening, the formulation of nursing diagnosis, the care of human responses to health and illness, and the evaluation of individual and family outcomes (ANA, 2004). The guiding principles for nurses to provide a continuum of services to individuals with I/DD across the lifespan include:

- Collaborative, comprehensive, and coordinated care;
- Cultural competence;
- Developmental appropriateness;
- Family-/youth-/person-centered care;
- Inclusiveness; and
- Normalization.

Each of these terms is defined in the glossary. Nurses in I/DD further provide services that incorporate system assessment, policy development and implementation, and quality assurance.

Nurses remain in this specialty because their passion is the care of individuals with I/DD. There are many challenges and rewards in this

The content in this appendix is not current and is of historical significance only.

field. Advances in science, especially in genetics and diagnostic technology, provide new insights and understanding of different conditions, their etiology, their trajectory, possible secondary conditions, and strategies for the management of the individual's health care so that quality of life can be and remain optimal. Learning about and caring for individuals with I/DD often enlighten and add meaning to one's nursing care.

Nurses who specialize in this field learn that we all are more alike than we are different. Nurses learn to appreciate an individual's strengths and assist the individual to cope and function with their limitations. Challenges include a multitude of healthcare problems that require many treatments or medications, uncertainty of the future because healthcare professionals do not know all there is to know about these conditions across the lifespan and especially in middle and late adulthood, and frustration with a society that thinks of persons with I/DD as different. There is a place for this nursing specialty and there always will be persons with I/DD who need to have someone care about and for their healthcare needs.

Professional Trends and Issues in I/DD

Currently, nurses in I/DD are involved through their practice and advocacy in a number of issues: predominant cultural concerns, early assessment and identification, inclusion in the school setting, adult health care, transition, self-advocacy and self-determination, employment, community living, managed care, and genetics. As nurses care for persons with I/DD and their families from diverse backgrounds, culturally competent methods of communication, care, and intervention must be developed and evaluated.

Nurses play a key role in the healthcare management of the person with I/DD throughout their life. Especially important is the transition from pediatric to adult healthcare services—ensuring that persons with I/DD living in a variety of residential settings, including the biological home, receive regular, quality health care, and that adolescents and adults with I/DD learn to advocate for themselves. New discoveries in the human genome have created vast opportunities for nurses to improve case identification, coordination, and referral; education;

The content in this appendix is not current and is of historical significance only.

identification, prevention, and management of primary and secondary disease conditions; and evaluation and follow-up of such conditions.

There is also a nursing shortage in this specialty. Efforts are being made in public and private agencies to increase salaries. Nursing organizations are developing continuing education and distance learning projects, as well as a core curriculum to assist nurses in learning more about I/DD and the needed nursing care. Nurses, across time, have contributed to the field by writing books, articles, and pamphlets, directing films, and producing Internet and distance learning products, to illustrate best practices and evidence-based care for nurses.

The content in this appendix is not current and is of historical significance only.

STANDARDS OF INTELLECTUAL AND DEVELOPMENTAL DISABILITIES (I/DD) NURSING PRACTICE

These standards provide direction for nurses specializing in this field, provide a foundation for evaluation of nursing practice, and represent the current level of knowledge and practice in that specialty. These standards apply to both the professional registered nurse and advanced practice registered nurse in I/DD. In the absence of the advanced practice registered nurse, the professional registered nurse assumes much, but not all, of the more comprehensive role of the advanced practice registered nurse. The authors recommend that the professional registered nurse level include nurses who are educationally prepared at the baccalaureate level. These standards apply to the nursing care of persons with I/DD of all ages, cultures, socioeconomic backgrounds, and medical diagnoses. Furthermore, these standards apply to any healthcare, education, residential, or community setting where individuals with I/DD might be.

Standards of practice for any specialty must be dynamic and reflect the current state of knowledge and practice. Standards of practice should be assessed along with other measures (e.g., educational degrees), documents [e.g., *Nursing's Social Policy Statement* (ANA 2003) and *Nursing: Scope and Standards of Practice* (ANA, 2004)], scientific evidence, and state nursing practice acts that provide guidelines for evaluating nursing practice. Standards of practice can be used:

- In practice for developing job position statements, performance evaluations, determining reimbursement ratings, and utilization review;

- In the development and validation of nursing theory and theory from related disciplines in relation to I/DD;

- In the development and testing of research questions;

- In the development, implementation, and evaluation of instruction to individuals and families by nurses or educational programs for groups of nurses, healthcare professionals, individuals with I/DD, their families, or the public;

The content in this appendix is not current and is of historical significance only.

- In the development of policy related to service, practice, and federal financing programs; and

- As clinical evidence for practice.

Each standard of practice and professional performance listed in this document has been standardized by the ANA (2004). The measurement criteria have been developed by the authors to represent quality practice and performance in the nursing care of individuals with I/DD.

STANDARDS OF PRACTICE OF INTELLECTUAL AND DEVELOPMENTAL DISABILITIES (I/DD) NURSING

STANDARD 1. ASSESSMENT
The registered nurse who specializes in I/DD collects comprehensive data pertinent to the patient's health or the situation.

Measurement Criteria
The registered nurse:

- Systematically collects data over time.

- Involves the individual with I/DD, family, other healthcare and interdisciplinary professionals and paraprofessionals, and the work and home environment, as appropriate, in obtaining comprehensive data. This may involve observation, interviewing, and the use of screening and assessment tools. Diagnostic tests may be used as part of the assessment process if the nurse has specific training in that area (e.g., developmental diagnostic testing).

- Prioritizes the data to be collected according to the immediate condition or anticipated needs, or the situation.

- Uses appropriate evidence-based assessment techniques and instruments in collecting pertinent data. This may include genetic studies, special serum screening (e.g., cystic fibrosis, Tay–Sachs, sickle-cell disease), nutritional needs and metabolic functioning, and any other condition-specific data.

- Uses analytical models and problem-solving tools that are appropriate for persons with I/DD.

- Synthesizes all data, information, and knowledge from the individual with I/DD, family members, the interdisciplinary team, and the individual's environment that is relevant to identify patterns and variances. This may involve data and information from the school, work site, or residential setting.

- Documents relevant data in a retrievable format.

The content in this appendix is not current and is of historical significance only.

Additional Measurement Criteria for the Advanced Practice Registered Nurse

The advanced practice registered nurse:

- Initiates and interprets diagnostic tests and procedures, relevant to the individual with I/DD's current status.

STANDARD 2. DIAGNOSIS
The registered nurse who specializes in I/DD analyzes the assessment data to determine the diagnoses or issues.

Measurement Criteria
The registered nurse:

- Identifies diagnoses or issues based on assessment data.

- Validates diagnoses or issues in partnership with the individual with I/DD, family, and members of the interdisciplinary team when possible and appropriate.

- Documents diagnoses or issues in a manner that facilitates the determination of the expected outcomes and plan.

Additional Measurement Criteria for the Advanced Practice Registered Nurse
The advanced practice registered nurse:

- Systematically compares and contrasts the history and clinical findings with normal and abnormal variations and developmental events in formulating differential diagnoses.

- Is aware that there may be specific values, ranges, and outcomes for a specific diagnosis (e.g., Down syndrome).

- Synthesizes all data and information collected during interview, examination, and diagnostic procedures (including developmental and supports assessment) to identify diagnoses.

- Serves as a consultant to the registered nurse and other staff in developing and maintaining competency in the diagnostic process.

Additional Measurement Criteria for the Nursing Role Specialty
The advanced practice registered nurse:

- Analyzes accessibility and availability of services, barriers to adequate health care, specific populations at high risk, health promotion needs for specific populations, and environmental hazards that may affect health.

STANDARD 3. OUTCOME IDENTIFICATION
The registered nurse who specializes in I/DD identifies expected outcomes for a plan to the patient or the situation.

Measurement Criteria

The registered nurse:

- Partners with the individual with I/DD, family, and members of the interdisciplinary team in formulating expected outcomes when possible and appropriate.

- Derives culturally appropriate expected outcomes from the diagnosis.

- Considers associated risks, benefits, and costs, current scientific evidence, and clinical expertise when formulating expected outcomes.

- Defines expected outcomes in terms of the individual with I/DD, his or her values, the values of the family members when appropriate, ethical and legal considerations, environment, or situation with such consideration as associated risks, benefits, and costs, and current scientific, ethical, and legal evidence.

- Includes a time estimate for attainment of expected outcomes.

- Develops expected outcomes that provide direction for continuity of care and person-centered care as appropriate.

- Modifies expected outcomes based on changes in status (i.e., health, social, living, economic, or legal) of the individual with I/DD or evidence of the situation.

- Documents expected outcomes as measurable goals.

Additional Measurement Criteria for the Advanced Practice Registered Nurse

The advanced practice registered nurse:

- Identifies expected outcomes that incorporate scientific evidence and are achievable through implementation of evidence-based practices.

The content in this appendix is not current and is of historical significance only.

- Identifies expected outcomes that incorporate cost and clinical effectiveness, legal and ethical boundaries, satisfaction and understanding, and consistency and continuity among the individual with I/DD, family members, healthcare providers, and members of the interdisciplinary team.

- Supports the use of clinical guidelines linked to positive patient outcomes.

Standard 4. Planning
The registered nurse who specializes in I/DD develops a plan that prescribes strategies and alternatives to attain expected outcomes.

Measurement Criteria
The registered nurse:

- Develops an individualized plan that is person-centered when appropriate, considering individual or situational characteristics (e.g., chronological and developmental age, culturally appropriate, and least restrictive environment).

- Develops the plan in collaboration with the individual with I/DD, family, others, and the interdisciplinary team, as appropriate.

- Includes strategies within the plan that address individual identified diagnoses or issues, which may include strategies for promotion and restoration of health and prevention of illness, injury, and disease.

- Provides for continuity within the plan.

- Incorporates an implementation pathway or timeline within the plan.

- Establishes the plan priorities with the individual with I/DD, family, others, and the interdisciplinary team as appropriate.

- Utilizes the plan to provide direction to other members of the healthcare and interdisciplinary team.

- Defines the plan to reflect current federal laws, statutes, rules and regulations, and standards.

- Integrates current trends and research affecting comprehensive care for the individual with I/DD in the planning process.

- Considers the economic impact of the plan.

- Uses standardized and person-first language or other recognized terminology to document the plan.

The content in this appendix is not current and is of historical significance only.

Additional Measurement Criteria for the Advanced Practice Nurse

The advanced practice registered nurse:

- Identifies assessment, screening and diagnostic strategies, and therapeutic interventions within the plan that reflect current evidence, including data, research, literature, and expert clinical knowledge.

- Selects or designs strategies to meet the multifaceted needs of complex individuals with I/DD.

- Includes the synthesis of the individual with I/DD's values and beliefs regarding nursing, medical, social, and educational therapies within the plan.

Additional Measurement Criteria for the Nursing Role Specialty

The registered nurse in a nursing role specialty:

- Participates in the design and development of interdisciplinary processes to address the situation or the issue.

- Contributes to the development and continuous improvement of organizational systems that support the planning process.

- Supports the integration of clinical, human, and financial resources to enhance and complete the decision-making and evaluation processes.

The advanced practice registered nurse in a nursing role specialty:

- Serves as a consultant to the registered nurse in plan development, priority setting, cost–benefit analysis, and identification of resources, as needed.

- In collaboration with the registered nurse, other members of the interdisciplinary team, and in partnership with the community, derives community-focused plans that are based on identified problems, conditions, or needs and that build on the strengths of the community.

- Develops plans that ensure continuity of care and minimize or eliminate gaps in and duplication of services.

STANDARD 5. IMPLEMENTATION
The registered nurse who specializes in I/DD implements the identified plan.

Measurement Criteria
The registered nurse:

- Implements the plan in a safe and timely manner.

- Documents implementation and any modifications, including changes or omissions, of the identified plan.

- Utilizes evidence-based interventions and treatments specific to the diagnosis or problem.

- Utilizes community resources and systems to implement the plan.

- Collaborates with nursing colleagues and others to implement the plan.

Additional Measurement Criteria for the Advanced Practice Registered Nurse
The advanced practice registered nurse:

- Facilitates utilization of systems and community resources to implement the plan.

- Supports collaboration with nursing colleagues and other members of the interdisciplinary team to implement the plan.

- Incorporates new knowledge and strategies to initiate change in nursing care practices if desired outcomes are not achieved.

Additional Measurement Criteria for the Nursing Role Specialty
The registered nurse in a nursing role specialty:

- Implements the plan using principles and concepts of project or systems management.

- Fosters organizational systems that support implementation of the plan.

STANDARD 5A: COORDINATION OF CARE
The registered nurse who specializes in I/DD coordinates delivery of care.

Measurement Criteria
The registered nurse:

- Coordinates implementation of the plan.
- Documents the coordination of the care.

Measurement Criteria for the Advanced Practice Registered Nurse
The advanced practice registered nurse:

- Provides leadership in the coordination of interdisciplinary health care for integrated delivery of patient care services.
- Synthesizes data and information to prescribe necessary system and community support measures, including environmental modifications.
- Coordinates system and community resources that enhance delivery of care across continuums.

Additional Measurement Criteria for the Nursing Role Specialty
The registered nurse in a nursing role specialty:

- Makes referrals to other disciplines as needed.
- Supervises or provides direction to ancillary and unlicensed personnel who provide health care to individuals with I/DD and their families.
- Keeps the individual and family (and direct care support professionals when present) informed about their health status.
- Keeps the individual and the family informed about healthcare resources that are available.
- Employs strategies to promote health in a safe and least restrictive environment in home and community settings.

STANDARD 5B: HEALTH TEACHING AND HEALTH PROMOTION
The registered nurse who specializes in I/DD employs strategies to promote health and a safe environment.

Measurement Criteria
The registered nurse:

- Provides health teaching that addresses such topics as healthy lifestyles, risk-reducing behaviors, developmental needs, activities of daily living, self-care concepts and skills, and preventive self-care.

- Uses health promotion and health teaching methods appropriate to the situation and the individual with I/DD's developmental level, learning needs, readiness, ability to learn, language preference, and culture.

- Seeks opportunities for feedback and evaluation of the effectiveness of the strategies used.

Additional Measurement Criteria for the Advanced Practice Registered Nurse
The advanced practice registered nurse:

- Synthesizes empirical evidence on risk behaviors, learning theories, behavioral change theories, motivational theories, epidemiology, and other related theories and frameworks when designing health information and patient education.

- Designs health information and patient education appropriate to the individual with I/DD's developmental level, learning needs, readiness to learn, and cultural values and beliefs.

- Evaluates health information resources, such as the Internet, within the area of practice for accuracy, readability, and comprehensibility to help individuals with I/DD, family, and other members of the interdisciplinary team access quality health information.

The content in this appendix is not current and is of historical significance only.

STANDARD 5C: CONSULTATION

The registered nurse and the advanced practice registered nurse who specializes in I/DD provide consultation to influence the identified plan, enhance the abilities of others, and effect change.

Measurement Criteria for the Advanced Practice Registered Nurse

The advanced practice registered nurse:

- Synthesizes clinical data, theoretical frameworks, and evidence when providing consultation.

- Facilitates the effectiveness of a consultation by involving the individual with I/DD and family in decision-making and negotiating role responsibilities.

- Communicates consultation recommendations that facilitate change.

Additional Measurement Criteria for the Nursing Role Specialty

The registered nurse in a nursing role specialty:

- Synthesizes data, information, theoretical frameworks, and evidence when providing consultation.

- Facilitates the effectiveness of a consultation by involving the stakeholders in the decision-making process.

- Communicates consultation recommendations that influence the identified plan, facilitate understanding by involving stakeholders, enhance the work of others, and effect change.

The advanced practice registered nurse in a nursing role specialty:

- Formulates and influences health and social policies that affect individuals with I/DD.

STANDARD 5D: PRESCRIPTIVE AUTHORITY AND TREATMENT

The advanced practice registered nurse who specializes in I/DD uses prescriptive authority, procedures, referrals, treatments, and therapies in accordance with state and federal laws and regulations.

Measurement Criteria for the Advanced Practice Registered Nurse

The advanced practice registered nurse:

- Prescribes evidenced-based treatments, therapies, and procedures, considering the individual with I/DD's comprehensive healthcare needs.

- Prescribes pharmacological agents based on a current knowledge of pharmacology and physiology.

- Prescribes specific pharmacological agents and/or treatments based on clinical indicators, the individual with I/DD's status and needs, and the results of diagnostic and laboratory tests.

- Evaluates therapeutic and potential adverse effects of pharmacological and nonpharmacological treatments.

- Provides individuals with I/DD and their families with information about intended effects and potential adverse effects of proposed prescriptive therapies.

- Provides information about costs as well as alternative treatments and procedures, as appropriate.

Additional Measurement Criteria for the Nursing Role Specialty

The advanced practice registered nurse in a nursing role specialty:

- Provides information and makes recommendations about changes needed in health policies, regulations, and laws affecting care provided by advanced practice registered nurses for individuals with I/DD.

STANDARD 6: EVALUATION
The registered nurse who specializes in I/DD evaluates progress toward attainment of outcomes.

Measurement Criteria
The registered nurse:

- Conducts a systematic, ongoing, and criterion-based evaluation of the outcomes in relation to the structures and processes pre-scribed by the plan and the indicated timeline.

- Includes the individual with I/DD and others involved in the care or situation in the evaluative process.

- Evaluates the effectiveness of the planned strategies in relation to individual with I/DD's responses and the attainment of the ex-pected outcomes.

- Documents the results of the evaluation.

- Using ongoing assessment data to revise the diagnoses, out-comes, the plan, and the implementation as needed.

- Disseminates the results to the individual with I/DD and others involved in the care or situation, as appropriate, in accordance with state and federal laws and regulations.

Additional Measurement Criteria for the Advanced Practice Registered Nurse
The advanced practice registered nurse:

- Evaluates the accuracy of the diagnoses and effectiveness of the interventions in relationship to the individual with I/DD's attain-ment of expected outcomes.

- Synthesizes the results of the evaluation analyses to determine the impact of the plan on the affected individuals with I/DD, families, groups, communities, and institutions.

- Uses the results of the evaluation analyses to make or recom-mend process or structural changes, including policy, procedure, or protocol documentation, as appropriate.

The content in this appendix is not current and is of historical significance only.

Additional Measurement Criteria for the Nursing Role Specialty

The registered nurse in a nursing role specialty:

- Uses the results of the evaluation analyses to make or recommend process or structural changes, including policy, procedure, or protocol documentation, as appropriate.

- Synthesizes the results of the evaluation analyses to determine the impact of the plan on the affected individuals with I/DD, families, groups, communities, institutions, networks, and organizations.

The content in this appendix is not current and is of historical significance only.

STANDARDS OF PROFESSIONAL PERFORMANCE OF INTELLECTUAL AND DEVELOPMENTAL DISABILITIES (I/DD) NURSING

STANDARD 7. QUALITY OF PRACTICE
The registered nurse who specializes in I/DD systematically enhances the quality and effectiveness of nursing practice.

Measurement Criteria

The registered nurse:

- Demonstrates quality by documenting the application of the nursing process in a responsible, accountable, and ethical manner.

- Uses the results of quality improvement activities to initiate changes in nursing practice and in the healthcare delivery system.

- Uses creativity and innovation in nursing practice to improve care delivery.

- Incorporates new knowledge to initiate changes in nursing practice if desired outcomes are not achieved.

- Participates in quality improvement activities. Such activities may include:

  - Identifying aspects of practice important for quality monitoring.

  - Using indicators developed to monitor quality and effectiveness of nursing practice.

  - Collecting data to monitor quality and effectiveness of nursing practice.

  - Analyzing quality data to identify opportunities for improving nursing practice.

  - Formulating recommendations to improve nursing practice or outcomes.

The content in this appendix is not current and is of historical significance only.

- Implementing activities to enhance the quality of nursing practice.

- Developing, implementing, and evaluating policies, procedures, and guidelines to improve the quality of practice.

- Participating on interdisciplinary teams to evaluate clinical care or health services.

- Participating in efforts to minimize costs and unnecessary duplication.

- Analyzing factors related to safety, satisfaction, effectiveness, and cost-benefit options.

- Analyzing organizational systems for barriers.

- Implementing processes to remove or decrease barriers within organizational systems.

Additional Measurement Criteria for the Advanced Practice Registered Nurse

The advanced practice registered nurse:

- Obtains and maintains professional certification if available in the area of expertise.

- Designs quality improvement initiatives.

- Implements initiatives to evaluate the need for change.

- Evaluates the practice environment and quality of nursing care rendered in relation to existing evidence, identifying opportunities for the generation and use of research.

Additional Measurement Criteria for the Nursing Role Specialty

The registered nurse in a nursing role specialty:

- Obtains and maintains professional certification if available in the area of expertise.

- Designs quality improvement initiatives.

- Implements initiatives to evaluate the need for change.

- Evaluates the practice environment in relation to existing evidence identifying opportunities for the generation and use of research in the care of individuals with I/DD.

- Evaluates nursing care delegated to other professionals, direct care support professionals, unlicensed assistive personnel, or the family and documents the effect of delegation on health outcomes.

- Participates in professional organizations which strive to improve the quality of nursing care and other services provided to individuals with I/DD and their families.

STANDARD 8. EDUCATION
The registered nurse who specializes in I/DD attains knowledge and competency that reflect current nursing practice.

Measurement Criteria
The registered nurse:

- Participates in ongoing educational activities related to appropriate knowledge bases and professional issues.

- Demonstrates a commitment to lifelong learning through self-reflection and inquiry to identify learning needs.

- Seeks experiences that reflect current practice to maintain skills and competence in clinical practice or role performance.

- Acquires knowledge and skills appropriate to the specialty area, practice setting, role, or situation.

- Maintains professional records that provide evidence of competency and lifelong learning.

- Seeks experiences and formal and independent learning activities to maintain and develop clinical and professional skills and knowledge.

Additional Measurement Criteria for the Advanced Practice Registered Nurse
The advanced practice registered nurse:

- Uses current healthcare research findings and other evidence to expand clinical knowledge, enhance role performance, and increase knowledge of professional issues.

Additional Measurement Criteria for the Nursing Role Specialty
The registered nurse in a nursing role specialty:

- Uses current research findings and other evidence related to the care of individuals with I/DD, to expand knowledge, enhance role performance, and increase knowledge of professional issues.

STANDARD 9. PROFESSIONAL PRACTICE EVALUATION

The registered nurse who specializes in I/DD evaluates one's own nursing practice in relation to professional practice standards and guidelines, relevant statutes, rules, and regulations.

Measurement Criteria

The registered nurse's practice reflects the application of knowledge of current practice standards, guidelines, statutes, rules, and regulations.

The registered nurse:

- Provides chronologically and developmentally age-appropriate care in a culturally and ethnically sensitive manner.

- Engages in self-evaluation of practice on a regular basis, identifying areas of strength, as well as areas in which professional development would be beneficial.

- Obtains informal feedback regarding one's own practice from individuals with I/DD, family members, peers, professional colleagues, and others, including direct care support professionals.

- Participates in systematic peer review as appropriate.

- Takes action to achieve goals identified during the evaluation process.

- Provides rationales for practice beliefs, decisions, and actions as part of the informal and formal evaluation processes.

Additional Measurement Criteria for the Advanced Practice Registered Nurse

The advanced practice registered nurse:

- Engages in a formal process, seeking feedback regarding one's own practice from individuals with I/DD, family members, peers, professional colleagues, and others, including direct care support professionals.

Additional Measurement Criteria for the Nursing Role Specialty

The registered nurse in a nursing role specialty:

- Engages in a formal process, seeking feedback regarding one's own practice from individuals with I/DD, family members, peers, professional colleagues, and others, including direct care support professionals.

STANDARD 10. COLLEGIALITY
The registered nurse who specializes in I/DD interacts with, and contributes to the professional development of, peers and colleagues.

Measurement Criteria
The registered nurse:

- Shares knowledge and skills with peers and colleagues as evidenced by such activities as patient care conferences or presentations at formal or informal meetings.

- Provides peers with feedback regarding their practice or role performance.

- Interacts with peers and colleagues to enhance one's own professional nursing practice or role performance.

- Maintains compassionate and caring relationships with peers and colleagues.

- Contributes to an environment that is conducive to the education of healthcare and other professionals that compose the interdisciplinary team.

- Contributes to a supportive and healthy work environment.

Additional Measurement Criteria for the Advanced Practice Registered Nurse
The advanced practice registered nurse:

- Models expert practice to interdisciplinary team members and healthcare consumers.

- Mentors other registered nurses and colleagues as appropriate.

- Participates with interdisciplinary teams that contribute to role development and advanced nursing practice and health care.

Additional Measurement Criteria for the Nursing Role Specialty

The registered nurse in a nursing role specialty:

- Participates on interdisciplinary teams that contribute to role development and, directly or indirectly, advance nursing practice and health services.

- Mentors other registered nurses, direct care support professionals, and colleagues as appropriate.

STANDARD 11. COLLABORATION

The registered nurse who specializes in I/DD collaborates with the individual with I/DD, family, and others in the conduct of nursing practice.

Measurement Criteria

The registered nurse:

- Communicates with the individual with I/DD, family, members of the interdisciplinary team, and healthcare providers regarding patient care and the nurse's role in the provision of that care.

- Collaborates in creating a documented plan, focused on outcomes and decisions related to care and delivery of services, that indicates communication with individuals with I/DD, families, and others.

- Partners with others to effect change and generate positive outcomes through knowledge of the individual with I/DD or situation.

- Documents referrals, including provisions for continuity of care.

Additional Measurement Criteria for the Advanced Practice Registered Nurse

The advanced practice registered nurse:

- Partners with other disciplines to enhance the care of individuals with I/DD through interdisciplinary activities, such as education, consultation, management, technological development, or research opportunities.

- Facilitates an interdisciplinary process with other members of the interdisciplinary and healthcare team.

- Documents plan of care communications, rationales for plan of care changes, and collaborative discussions to improve the care of individuals with I/DD.

The content in this appendix is not current and is of historical significance only.

Additional Measurement Criteria for the Nursing Role Specialty

The registered nurse in a nursing role specialty:

- Partners with others to enhance health care and, ultimately, care of the individual with I/DD, through interdisciplinary activities such as education, consultation, management, technological development, or research opportunities.

- Documents plans, communications, rationales for plan changes, and collaborative discussions.

- Collaborates with the individual with I/DD and family or significant others, and supports the efforts of patients and families to make appropriate decisions about utilization of resources.

The advanced practice registered nurse in a nursing role specialty:

- Participates with other interdisciplinary administrative team members in policy-making and in overall agency and community planning, implementation, and evaluation of services to and programs for individuals with I/DD.

Standard 12. Ethics
The registered nurse who specializes in I/DD integrates ethical provisions in all areas of practice.

Measurement Criteria
The registered nurse:

- Uses *Code of Ethics for Nurses with Interpretive Statements* (ANA 2001) to guide practice.
- Delivers care in a manner that preserves and protects the autonomy, dignity, and rights of individuals with I/DD.
- Maintains confidentiality of the individual with I/DD within legal and regulatory parameters.
- Serves as an advocate for the individual with I/DD by assisting them in developing skills for self-advocacy.
- Maintains a therapeutic and professional patient–nurse relationship with appropriate professional role boundaries.
- Demonstrates a commitment to practicing self-care, managing stress, and connecting with self and others.
- Contributes to resolving ethical issues of individuals with I/DD, colleagues, or systems as evidenced in such activities as participating on ethics committees.
- Reports illegal, incompetent, or impaired practices.

Additional Measurement Criteria for the Advanced Practice Registered Nurse
The advanced practice registered nurse:

- Informs the individual with I/DD and family members of the risks, benefits, and outcomes of healthcare regimens.
- Participates in interdisciplinary teams that address ethical risks, benefits, and outcomes.

The content in this appendix is not current and is of historical significance only.

Additional Measurement Criteria for the Nursing Role Specialty

The registered nurse in a nursing role specialty:

- Participates on interdisciplinary teams that address ethical risks, benefits, and outcomes.

- Informs administrators or others of the risks, benefits, and outcomes of programs and decisions that affect healthcare delivery.

- Respects the individual with I/DD's right to self-determination and includes the individual in decisions unless the individual's incapacity to participate in a specific decision is demonstrated. Family or a legally designated guardian is included in decision-making, or makes the decision as a surrogate decision-maker if legally required.

- Acts as an advocate for individuals with I/DD and their families when appropriate.

- Facilitates the individual with I/DD's self-determination in all healthcare settings.

- Refers the individual with I/DD to a qualified advocate when appropriate.

- Works to prevent and promptly respond to suspicion or evidence of abuse or exploitation, and reports the abuse to appropriate authorities.

- Identifies a surrogate for healthcare decisions in lieu of a formal guardianship process, when appropriate and in accordance with local or state statutes.

- Advocates for the individual with I/DD's self-determination when in conflict with the surrogate decision-maker.

- Assists in identifying the most appropriate living arrangements for the individual with I/DD in the least restrictive environment.

- Contributes to the educational program recommendations and advocates for the least restrictive environment to maximize the individual with I/DD's potential.

- Contributes to the life plan and advocates for the most appropriate employment situation. The nurse assists in identifying reasonable accommodations to maximize the individual with I/DD's performance and satisfaction with chosen employment.

- Serves as an advocate to ensure that individuals with I/DD have access to health care that provides continuity and is provided by a practitioner competent to manage the health concerns of individuals with I/DD.

- Facilitates the individual with I/DD's expression of sexuality in a manner that is consistent with the individual's native culture, religious upbringing, family values, and level of maturity, and provides counseling as appropriate. The nurse contributes to an environment that protects the individual with I/DD from sexual exploitation at home, school, work, and in the community.

- Assists in the referral process for local, state, regional, and federal assistance programs.

The content in this appendix is not current and is of historical significance only.

STANDARD 13. RESEARCH
The registered nurse who specializes in I/DD integrates research findings into practice.

Measurement Criteria

The registered nurse:

- Uses the best available evidence, including research findings, to guide practice decisions.

- Actively participates in research activities at various levels appropriate to the nurse's level of education and position. Such activities may include:

  - Identifying clinical problems specific to nursing research (patient care and nursing practice).

  - Participating in data collection (surveys, pilot projects, formal studies).

  - Participating in a formal committee or program.

  - Sharing research activities and findings with peers and others.

  - Conducting research.

  - Critically analyzing and interpreting research for application to practice.

  - Using research findings in the development of policies, procedures, and standards of practice in patient care.

  - Incorporating research as a basis for learning.

Additional Measurement Criteria for the Advanced Practice Registered Nurse

The advanced practice registered nurse:

- Contributes to nursing knowledge by conducting or synthesizing research that discovers, examines, and evaluates knowledge, theories, criteria, and creative approaches to improve healthcare practice.

- Formally disseminates research findings through activities such as presentations, publications, consultation, and journal clubs.

Additional Measurement Criteria for the Nursing Role Specialty

The registered nurse in a nursing role specialty:

- Contributes to nursing knowledge in the field of I/DD by conducting or synthesizing research that discovers, examines, and evaluates knowledge, theories, criteria, and creative approaches to improve healthcare practice and lives of individuals with I/DD.

- Participates in human subject protection activities as appropriate and is particularly cognizant of the vulnerability and exploitation of individuals with I/DD.

- Formally disseminates research findings through activities such as presentations, publications, consultation, interdisciplinary team meetings, and journal clubs.

The content in this appendix is not current and is of historical significance only.

STANDARD 14. RESOURCE UTILIZATION
The registered nurse specializing in I/DD considers factors related to safety, effectiveness, cost, and impact on practice in the planning and delivery of nursing services to individuals with I/DD.

Measurement Criteria
The registered nurse:

- Evaluates factors, such as safety, effectiveness, availability, cost and benefits, efficiencies, and impact on practice when choosing practice options that would result in the same expected outcome.

- Assists the individual with I/DD, family, or significant others in identifying and securing appropriate and available services to address health-related needs.

- Assigns or delegates tasks based on the needs and condition of the individual with I/DD, potential for hardship, stability of the individual with I/DD's condition, complexity of the task, and predictability of the outcome.

- Assists the individual with I/DD and family in becoming informed consumers about the options, costs, risks, and benefits of treatment and care.

Additional Measurement Criteria for the Advanced Practice Registered Nurse
The advanced practice registered nurse:

- Uses organizational and community resources to formulate interdisciplinary plans of care.

- Develops innovative solutions for patient care problems that address effective resource utilization and maintenance of quality.

- Develops evaluation strategies to demonstrate cost effectiveness, cost benefit, and efficiency factors associated with nursing practice.

The content in this appendix is not current and is of historical significance only.

Additional Measurement Criteria for the Nursing Role Specialty

The registered nurse in a nursing role specialty:

- Develops innovative solutions and applies strategies to obtain appropriate resources for nursing initiatives.

- Secures organizational resources to ensure a work environment conducive to completing the identified plan and outcomes.

- Develops evaluation methods to measure safety and effectiveness for interventions and outcomes.

- Promotes activities that assist others, as appropriate, in becoming informed about costs, risks, and benefits of care, or of the plan and solution.

Standard 15. Leadership
The nurse who specializes in I/DD provides leadership in the professional practice setting and the profession.

Measurement Criteria

The registered nurse:

- Engages in teamwork as a team player and a team builder.

- Works to create and maintain healthy work environments in local, regional, national, or international communities.

- Displays the ability to define a clear vision, the associated goals, and a plan to implement and measure progress.

- Demonstrates a commitment to continuous, lifelong learning for self and others.

- Teaches others to succeed by mentoring and other strategies.

- Exhibits creativity and flexibility through times of change.

- Demonstrates energy, excitement, and a passion for quality work.

- Willingly accepts mistakes by self and others, thereby creating a culture in which risk-taking is not only safe, but expected.

- Inspires loyalty through valuing of people as the most precious asset in an organization.

- Directs the coordination of care across settings and among caregivers, including oversight of licensed and unlicensed personnel, including direct care support professionals, in any assigned or delegated tasks.

- Serves in key roles in the work setting by participating on committees, councils, and administrative teams.

- Promotes advancement of the profession through participation in professional nursing and interdisciplinary organizations.

Additional Measurement Criteria for the Advanced Practice Registered Nurse

The advanced practice registered nurse:

- Works to influence decision-making bodies to improve the care of individuals with I/DD.

- Provides direction to enhance the effectiveness of the healthcare team.

- Initiates and revises protocols or guidelines to reflect evidence-based practice, to reflect accepted changes in care management, or to address emerging problems.

- Promotes communication of information and advancement of the profession through writing, publishing, and presentations for professional or lay audiences.

- Designs innovations to effect change in practice and improve health outcomes.

Additional Measurement Criteria for the Nursing Role Specialty

The registered nurse in a nursing role specialty:

- Works to influence decision-making bodies to improve patient care, health services, and policies as they affect individuals with I/DD.

- Promotes communication of information and advancement of the profession as it relates to nursing and the field of I/DD through writing, publishing, and presentations for professional or lay audiences.

- Designs innovations to effect change in practice and outcomes.

- Provides direction to enhance the effectiveness of the inter-disciplinary team.

GLOSSARY

Collaborative care. Care based on interdisciplinary problem-solving in which there is respect for the perspectives, abilities, knowledge, and experiences of each person who is involved in making decisions that affect an individual's health, education, or vocational goals and programs.

Comprehensive care. Care that integrates health (primary, secondary, and tertiary levels) and social/family support programs with educational or vocational services.

Coordinated care. Care that facilitates access to needed resources and services and promotes continuity of care among multiple providers and diverse service systems. Work is done collaboratively with the individual and family members to achieve mutually agreed upon goals. Timeliness, appropriateness, and completeness of care are central to this concept.

Cultural competence. Care that respects, honors, and incorporates beliefs, norms, attitudes, and life practices of individuals and their families.

Developmentally appropriate care. Care focused on the unique needs of individuals to promote the developmental skills and independence consistent with the individual's present functional abilities rather than chronological age.

Developmental screening. Assessing a person's global or specific domains of development for evidence of developmental deviation. The results of screening are not diagnostic, and if the results are suspicious they must be repeated within a short period. If developmental delay is suspected after repeated screening, the person should be referred for diagnosis and appropriate treatment and intervention.

Early intervention. The provision of health, social, and educational services in an interdisciplinary setting for children from birth to 3 years of age at risk for or diagnosed with I/DD.

Family-centered care. Care to individuals in need of special services (e.g., therapies, rehabilitation, adaptive equipment) that is provided within the context of their family. The strengths, individuality, and diversity of each family are acknowledged and valued. The cornerstone of family-centered care is a partnership between the family and the professionals.

Inclusion. Integration of all persons, regardless of special needs and disabilities or the environment (e.g., school, community, etc.), with typical peers in the least restrictive setting. Innovative programs geared to the individual's strengths and capabilities must be provided.

Individualized education plan (IEP). An annual educational program plan and goals that are jointly determined by the school teachers, therapists, school nurse, and parents of the school-aged child with I/DD and members of their support system. The IEP includes all developmental and academic testing results, the child's health status, and the child's strengths and weaknesses, as well as transition plans. This plan may include vocational goals beginning at age 14.

Individualized family service plan (IFSP). An annual family service plan that includes goals and interventions for the entire family of a child, birth to 3 years diagnosed with or at risk for I/DD. The IFSP includes the child's strengths and weaknesses, the results of developmental testing in all areas of adaptive living, family needs, the identification of community resources, and plans for transition to the school setting. This plan is devised by the interdisciplinary team and the parents of the child with I/DD and members of their support system.

Individualized plan for employment (IPE). An annual work or habilitation plan, usually completed for adults with I/DD, that includes goals and interventions as determined by the individual, their family, and the interdisciplinary team at the individual's place of employment or residence. The IPE includes all developmental, adaptive skill levels, habilitative training and skill levels, and the individual's strengths and weaknesses, which are summarized into a plan.

Individualized transition plan (ITP). An annual transition plan, to begin when the adolescent with I/DD reaches 14 to 16 years of age, which includes goals and interventions as determined by the individual, his or her family, and the interdisciplinary team for the transition to adulthood. The ITP includes the individual's health, developmental, adaptive skill levels, strengths and weaknesses, and goals for a successful transition into adulthood that incorporates all aspects of the individual's life.

Interdisciplinary team. A group of professionals with varied and specialized backgrounds who work with the individual and family to make decisions about all aspects of the individual with I/DD's life and includes health, education, and vocational needs. This planning should be person centered. The membership of the interdisciplinary team should be determined by the type of expertise needed to meet the individual's needs.

Least restrictive environment. Identification of the environment that offers the person with I/DD the least amount of restriction from carrying out their activities of daily living.

Normalization. Providing a supportive environment for persons with I/DD to make decisions regarding activities of daily living and to live as close as possible to the norms and patterns in the mainstream of the society in which they reside.

Nursing. The protection, promotion, and optimization of health and abilities, prevention of illness and injury, alleviation of suffering through the diagnosis and treatment of human response, and advocacy in the care of individuals, families, communities, and populations (ANA, 2003).

Person-centered (youth-centered) care. Care that is centered around the wishes of the individual with I/DD after the individual and their family are fully informed of the knowledge and options available in regards to their care.

Scope of practice. The art and science or the totality of the practice of nursing.

Standard. Authoritative statements by which the nursing profession describes responsibilities for which its practitioners are accountable. These standards reflect the values and priorities of the profession and provide direction for nursing practice and a framework for the evaluation of practice. Standards define the nursing profession's accountability to the public and the client outcomes for which nurses are responsible (ANA, 1991).

Standards of practice. Authoritative statements that encompass the minimal competency level of nursing care and involve the process of assessment, diagnosis, outcomes identification, planning, implementation, and evaluation.

Standards of professional performance. Authoritative statements that encompass the minimal competency level of professional performance and involve the functions of quality of practice, education, professional practice evaluation, collegiality, collaboration, ethics, research, resource utilization, and leadership.

The content in this appendix is not current and is of historical significance only.

REFERENCES

Aggen, R. L., M. D. DeGennaro, L. Fox, J. E. Hahn, B. A. Logan, and L. VonFumetti. 1995. *Standards of developmental disabilities nursing practice.* Eugene, OR: Developmental Disabilities Nurses Association.

Aggen, R. L., and N. J. Moore. 1984. *Standards of nursing practice in mental retardation/developmental disabilities.* Albany: New York State Office of Mental Retardation and Developmental Disabilities.

American Nurses Association (ANA). 2004. *Nursing: Scope and standards of practice.* Washington, DC: nursesbooks.org.

———. 2003. *Nursing's social policy statement.* 2nd ed. Washington, DC: nursesbooks.org.

———. 2001. *Code of ethics for nurses with interpretive statements.* Washington, DC: American Nurses Publishing.

———. 1999. *Scope and standards of public health nursing practice.* Washington, DC: American Nurses Publishing.

———. 1991. *Standards of clinical nursing practice.* Washington, DC: American Nurses Publishing.

American Psychiatric Nurses Association, International Society of Psychiatric–Mental Health Nurses, and American Nurses Association. 2000. *Scope and standards of psychiatric-mental health nursing practice.* Washington, DC: American Nurses Publishing.

Asch, A. 2001. Disability, bioethics, and human rights. In *Handbook of disability studies,* ed. G. L. Albrecht, K. D. Seelman, and M. Bury. Thousand Oaks, CA: Sage.

Austin, J., M. Challela, C. Huber, W. Sciarillo, and C. Stade. 1987. *Standards for the clinical advanced practice registered nurse in developmental disabilities/handicapping conditions.* Washington, DC: American Association of University Affiliated Programs.

Burling, S. 2002. Penn hospital to limit its care in futile cases. *Philadelphia Inquirer*, November 4, p. A1.

Colorado Collective for Medical Decisions. 1999. *Neonatal guidelines.* Denver: Author.

Consensus Committee. 1993. *National standards of nursing practice for early intervention services.* Lexington: University of Kentucky, College of Nursing.

———. 1994. *Standards of nursing practice for the care of children and adolescents with special health and developmental needs.* Vienna, VA: National Maternal and Child Health Clearinghouse.

Developmental Disabilities Assistance and Bill of Rights Act of 2000. 2000. Pub L. No. 106-402, 114 Stat. 1678.

Haynes, U. 1968. *Guidelines for nursing standards in residential centers for the mentally retarded.* Washington, DC: United Cerebral Palsy Association.

Igoe, J. B., P. Green, H. Heim, M. Licata, G. P. MacDonough, and B. A. McHugh. 1980. *School nurses working with handicapped children.* Kansas City, MO: American Nurses Association.

International Society of Nurses in Genetics, Inc., and American Nurses Association. 1998. *Statement on the scope and standards of genetics clinical nursing practice.* Washington, DC: American Nurses Publishing.

Luckasson, R., S., et al. 2002. *Mental retardation: Definition, classification, and systems of supports.* 10th ed. Washington, DC: American Association on Mental Retardation.

National Association of School Nurses and American Nurses Association. 2001. *Scope and standards of professional school nursing practice.* Washington, DC: American Nurses Publishing.

Nehring, W. M. 1999. *A history of nursing in the field of mental retardation and developmental disabilities.* Washington, DC: American Association on Mental Retardation.

Nerney, T. 2000. *This is freedom.* White paper delivered to AAMR 12th Annual Meeting, Washington, DC Retrieved December 8, 2003 from URL: http://www.aamr.org/Reading_Room/pdf/nerney_whitepaper.pdf

———. 2003. The American experience. *Learning Disability Practice* 6, no. 3:20–2.

Nehring, W. M., S. P. Roth, D. Natvig, J. S. Morse, T. Savage, and M. Krajicek. 1998. *Statement on the scope and standards for the nurse who specializes in developmental disabilities and/or mental retardation.* Washington, DC: American Nurses Association and American Association on Mental Retardation.

Roth, S. P., and J. S. Morse, J. S., eds. 1994. *A life-span approach to nursing care for individuals with developmental disabilities.* Baltimore: Brookes.

Society of Pediatric Nurses and American Nurses Association. 2003. *Scope and standards of pediatric nursing practice.* Washington, DC: American Nurses Publishing.

U.S. Public Health Service. 2002. *Closing the gap: A national blueprint for improving the health of individuals with mental retardation.* Report of the Surgeon General's conference on health disparities and mental retardation. Washington, DC: Author.

Williams, G. 2001. Theorizing disability. In *Handbook of disability studies,* ed. G. L. Albrecht, K. D. Seelman, M. Bury. Thousand Oaks, CA: Sage.

Index

as focus of care and practice, 2, 4, 9,
25, 31–32, 109, 118
health teaching and promotion and,
56, 57
as healthcare consumers, 76
leadership and, 71, 72
outcomes identification and, 47, 48
planning and, 49, 50
quality of practice and, 67, 68
See also Healthcare consumers

Family-centered care, defined, 84,
155–156

Financial issues. *See* Cost and economic
controls

The Future of Disability in America, 30

G

Genetic and genomic advances, IDD and,
36–37, 113

*The Guidelines for Nursing Standards in
Residential Centers for the Mentally
Retarded*, 5, 110

H

Haynes, Una H., 24

Healing in IDDN practice, 9, 33, 35

Health (defined), 84

Health teaching and promotion in IDDN
practice, 15
competencies involving, 56–57
Standard of Practice, 56–57
[2004], 132
See also Promotive IDDN practice

Healthcare, defined, 9

Healthcare consumers, 1, 3, 9, 20, 76, 84
interprofessional team for, 26
safety of, 29
See also Families

Healthcare home/medical home, 37, 86

Healthcare providers (defined), 84

Holistic focus of nursing practice, 33

I

IASSID. *See* International Association
for the Scientific Study of Intellectual
Disability (IASSID)

IDD. *See* Intellectual and developmental
disabilities (IDD)

IDDN. *See* Intellectual and
developmental disabilities nursing
(IDDN)

IEP. *See* Individualized education plan
(IEP)

IFSP. *See* Individualized family service
plan (IFSP)

Illness (defined), 84

Implementation in IDDN practice
competencies involving, 52–53
defined, 85
delegation and, 85
as nursing process step, 7–8, 14, 15, 31
Standard of Practice, 52–53
[2004], 130

Inclusion (defined), 85, 156

Individualization of IDDN practice, 9, 32

Individualized education plan (IEP)
defined, 85, 156

Individualized family service plan (IFSP)
defined, 85, 156

Individualized plan for employment (IPE)
defined, 85, 156

Individualized transition plan (ITP)
defined, 85–86, 156

Information (defined), 86

Institute of Medicine (IOM)
on competence evaluation, 19–20
on healthy work environments, 12
quality of care and practice and,
29–31

Institutional policies and procedures
as level in regulation of nursing, 11, 13

theory and, 24

work environments and, 12

See also Critical thinking, analysis, and synthesis; Education of IDD nurses; Evidence-based practice and research

Knowledge (defined), 86

L

Laws, statutes, and regulations in IDDN practice
advanced practice and, 28
advocacy and, 28

Leadership in IDDN practice, 16
competencies involving, 71–72
quality of practice and, 30
Standard of Professional Performance, 71–72
[2004], 153–154
transformational leadership, 11, 12
work environments and, 11, 12, 30

Learning in professional nursing, competence and, 18

Least restrictive environment, defined, 86, 157

Legal issues. *See* Laws, statutes, and regulations

Licensing and licensure in IDDN practice, 26–28
IDD registered nurses, 20–22
jurisdictions, 13

A Life-Span Approach to Nursing Care for Individuals with Developmental Disabilities, 6, 110

M

Magnet Recognition Program (ANCC) on healthy work environments, 11–12

Maternal and Child Health Bureau, 22

McNelly, Pat, 24

Measurement criteria for IDDN practice

[2004]
assessment, 123–124
collaboration, 144–145
collegiality, 142–143
consultation, 133
coordination of care, 131
diagnosis, 125
education, 140
ethics, 146–148
evaluation, 135–136
health teaching and health promotion, 132
implementation, 130
leadership, 153–154
outcomes identification, 126–127
planning, 128–129
prescriptive authority and treatment, 134
professional practice evaluation, 141
quality of practice, 137–139
research, 149–150
resource utilization, 151–152
See also Competencies for nursing standards

Medical errors. *See* Errors

Medical home/healthcare home, 37, 86

Mental retardation, defined, 2, 3, 107

Mental Retardation Division, Department of Health, Education, and Welfare, 5, 110

Mentoring in IDDN practice, 19

Midwifery. *See* Certified nurse midwives (CNM)

Mimosa Project, 24

Model of Professional Nursing Practice Regulation, 12–14

Models and frameworks in IDDN
of caring, 35–37
Consensus Model for APRN Regulation: Licensure, Accreditation, Certification & Education, 28
medical home/healthcare home, 37
of nursing practice regulation, 12–14
nursing process, 7–8

See also Nursing process; Theories and theory in nursing

Multidisciplinary healthcare. *See* Interprofessional health care

N

National Academies of Sciences, 29

National Council of State Boards of Nursing, 18

National licensing exam (NCLEX), 19, 21

NCAST. *See* Nursing Child Assessment Satellite Training (NCAST) Scales

NCLEX. *See* National licensing exam (NCLEX)

Newborns, with IDD, 4, 109

Nightingale, Florence, 23

Normalization, defined, 86, 157

Nursesbooks.org, xi

Nursing: Scope and Standards of Practice (ANA), xiii

Nursing activities, 3, 15, 24, 35

Nursing care, IDD and, 4, 111

Nursing care standards. *See* Standards of Practice

Nursing Child Assessment Satellite Training (NCAST) Scales, 24

Nursing competence. *See* Competence and competencies

Nursing (defined), 2, 86, 106–108, 157
    See also Nursing practice

Nursing Division of the American Association on Mental Retardation, 6, 111, 115

Nursing education
    progression of, 29
    See also Education of IDD nurses

Nursing interventions. *See* Interventions

Nursing judgments. *See* Judgments

Nursing models. *See* Models and frameworks in IDD

Nursing practice
    defined, 87
    IDDN (*See* Intellectual and developmental disabilities nursing)

Nursing process, 7–8
    defined, 87
    individualized care and, 10
    science of nursing and, 31, 111–114
    Standards of Practice and, 13
    See also Standards of Practice; Specific standards

Nursing profession, IDDN
    commitment to, 37–38, 118–119
    trends and issues, 38–39, 119–120

Nursing professional organizations. *See* Organizations and IDDN practice; Specific organizations

Nursing Role Specialty [2004]
    measurement criteria, 125, 129, 130, 131, 133, 134, 136, 138, 140, 141, 143, 145, 147, 150, 152, 154
    See also Specialty nursing practice

Nursing shortage, 39, 120

Nursing standards
    development and function of IDD, 7
    See also Standards of Professional Nursing Practice for IDDN

Nursing's Social Policy Statement: The Essence of the Profession (ANA), 2, 25, xiii

O

Organizational policies and procedures, as level in regulation of nursing, 11

Organizations and IDDN practice
    and healthy work environments, 11, 12, 29
    interdisciplinary, 21
    responsibilities, 12, 21

Outcomes identification in IDDN practice
    competencies involving, 47–48
    evidence-based practice and research